End of
INJURY

Other books by Ted Gambordella:

Seven Days to Self-Defense

How to Develop a Perfect Body in Thirty Minutes a Day

The Complete Book of Karate Weapons

Full Contact Karate—with "The Golden Greek"

End of
INJURY

Theodore L. Gambordella, Ph. D.

Contemporary Books, Inc.
Chicago

Library of Congress Cataloging in Publication Data

Gambordella, Theodore L
   End of injury.

   Includes index.
   1. Sports—Training.   2. Physical fitness.
3. Sports—Accidents and injuries—Prevention.
I. Title.
GV711.5.G35   617'.1027   80-10465
ISBN 0-8092-7085-4
ISBN 0-8092-7084-6 pbk.

Copyright © 1980 by Theodore L. Gambordella
All rights reserved
Published by Contemporary Books, Inc.
180 North Michigan Avenue, Chicago, Illinois 60601
Manufactured in the United States of America
Library of Congress Catalog Card Number: 80-10465
International Standard Book Number: 0-8092-7085-4 (cloth)
                                     0-8092-7084-6 (paper)

Published simultaneously in Canada by
Beaverbooks
953 Dillingham Road
Pickering, Ontario L1W 1Z7
Canada

CONTENTS

INTRODUCTION

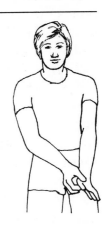

I wrote this book because every year there are thousands of preventable injuries to professional, collegiate, and amateur athletes. It seems that in America most people do not worry about something until it's too late. Take illness for example. We spend billions in alleviating the symptoms of the illness—medicine to stop the drippy nose, ease the pain, relieve the pressure, etc. But we spend very little to prevent the body from becoming ill. Our country spends billions of dollars on medical research to cure illness but only a pittance on research to prevent the illness. The same thing holds true for sports and sport-related injuries.

Every year thousands of athletes fall down and break or tear a part of their bodies. Every year thousands of athletes get hit in the ribs or abdomen and break bones or injure internal organs. Every day someone makes a mistake while playing and finds himself injured, perhaps permanently because no one ever told him how to *PREVENT ATHLETIC INJURIES*. This book does just that—gives easy to follow, proven techniques for the prevention of athletic injuries. Of course this book will not make you a Superman or prevent all injuries. What it will do is provide alternatives by teaching you how to roll instead of break, to stretch instead of tear, and to absorb impacts instead of crushing your body.

This book is based on three logical assumptions.

1. There are only three ways that an injury can occur and there are proven

techniques that can help prevent these injuries:

a. Stretching or flexibility related injuries (pulling or tearing muscles from overstretching the muscles, tendons, or ligaments). Solution: Following a complete stretching program.

b. Falling and breaking bones, or injuring muscles, joints, and the body in general. Solution: Using proper falling techniques.

c. Getting hit (contact that breaks bones, injures muscle). Solution: Practicing Ki (breath, muscle, and mind control all used simultaneously).

2. A relaxed athlete is able to perform better and is less likely to be injured. When you are upset, your body overreacts and your mind becomes confused so that you are not able to perform at your top level.

3. Size and strength can be overcome by the use of balance points and leverage. A child can balance a 400 pound refrigerator on one corner if he maintains the balance. It took you two years to learn to walk and your balance is conditional upon the cooperation of your entire body (the eyes, inner ears, toes, arms, hips, etc.). Force can be applied in only one direction, and if you learn to utilize the techniques of balance and leverage in this book you can easily maneuver and manipulate a much larger and stronger opponent.

If you will study this book with an open mind, begin to practice the techniques and exercises found herein, in a few short weeks you will begin to understand and to utilize the techniques found in it. Your ability to concentrate will greatly improve, your skills will sharpen, and your mind will become stronger. You will have a much greater ability to withstand blows and hits that would injure most people; you will improve your performance by the use of balance points, concentration, and mind control.

Why the Techniques Found in This Book Will Work

The techniques found in this book come primarily from martial art techniques. Many people are prejudiced against martial arts; in America the martial arts are not respected as they are in the Orient. Many practitioners of the martial arts in America profess themselves to be better than they are; even when they have little knowledge and are poor in technique, they go around telling everyone that they are the greatest. Only one person can be the greatest. So such persons usually find themselves in compromising situations such as breaking their hands trying to break bricks, or getting punched out by a "weaker" opponent. But this does not mean that the techniques and the art form that they have learned are not effective. It only means that they are not effective in using them. A gun will certainly kill you, but first you have to hit the person with the bullet. So martial art techniques are definitely effective *if* the person doing them hits the target with the right technique.

The martial arts are just that—art forms. As such they are beautiful to watch and tend to become a way of life with the true practitioners. They are techniques that can be enjoyed and practiced for benefit by anyone, just as any great work of art can be enjoyed by all viewers.

The techniques found in this book do not just come from Karate, which is what many people think of when they hear the words martial arts, but they come from Judo, Jujitsu, Kung Fu, Aikido, Kendo, Zen, Yoga, and even psychology and ballet. Techniques that can be applicable to all forms of sports have been utilized in this manual for the mutual benefit of the players and the fans. No one wants to get hurt or see a player get hurt, and everyone wants maximum performance, a positive attitude, and a stronger mind.

Let us examine the facts:

1. There is no better way in the world to learn how to fall without receiving an injury than to practice Judo falling techniques.

2. The most flexible people in the world are ballet dancers and those who practice Karate. The stretches taken from these two arts will enable you to become as flexible as you wish.

3. There is only one art form in the world that teaches you how to get hit without getting injured: Jujitsu, and it does not require any magical mystical powers. It is simply breath, muscle, and mind control all put together to form a new identity called Ki. (Just like the various pieces of metal are all put together and form a new machine called a car.)

4. There is no better form of exercise to develop powers of concentration and mind control than techniques of meditation taken from Zen and Yoga.

5. Aikido is a 2,000-year-old art form that enables one to overcome the largest of opponents with the minimal amount of effort by the use of balance points and leverage.

6. Breathing is both necessary to sustain life and vital in athletic performance, in relaxation, and in concentration. If you don't believe me, hold your breath for a week, or try to sleep while breathing 70 times a minute. The best techniques of breath control in the world come from Yoga and its exercises.

7. The most powerful method ever developed of striking or hitting another person or thing comes from Karate techniques of weight shifting and striking. (Ever try to break a brick?)

8. Techniques of one sport can be applied effectively to other sports.

So please do not find yourself being prejudiced against techniques found in this book before you even try them. They are the most effective means man has ever found to do the things described; if you will use them in your sport, you can improve your performance, develop a positive mental attitude, and prevent most injuries. Keep an open mind; practice them and apply them in any way you wish. Adapt them to your style and use them at your discretion, but use them and you and your sport will benefit greatly.

End of
INJURY

CHAPTER 1

Flexibility

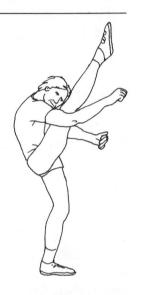

The importance of flexibility in preventing athletic injuries and improving performance cannot be overemphasized. The flexibility of the athlete is vital in the reduction of leg injuries, the increase of the player's own body control, and the improvement of performance due to the increase of mobility and coordination. Such injuries as a pulled hamstring, a pulled groin, or a sprained ankle are much less likely to occur when the athlete has adequate flexibility. In fact, many professional teams now employ a full time flexibility coach to help assure full performance and to reduce flexibility related injuries.

There is a vast difference between a muscle being "stretched" and a "limber" muscle. Once a muscle has been truly "stretched" it will tend to remain so

over a great period of time. It is like folding a piece of paper; once the fold has been made, the paper will always have a crease in it. So once a muscle has been stretched, it will always have the tendency to remain so. A muscle that has only been limbered up is one that will quickly snap back to its shorter state, thereby increasing the chances of a flexibility related injury.

The proper method for performing a stretching program is to take your time and allow the muscles to gradually lengthen as you bend, not bounce or jerk in your movements. It is virtually impossible to loosen up and truly stretch a muscle in 10 seconds (as you often see athletes try to do when the coach calls them off the bench into the game).

If the athlete goes into the game cold,

or not fully limber or stretched, then he is going to have to use a few minutes of the actual game time to get loose enough for his top performance. This could mean giving up a first down, missing a block or a tackle, blowing a shot, etc. So the athlete should strive to stay stretched on the sidelines by doing a few simple stretches while he is sitting on the bench, standing on the sidelines, or even waiting between plays.

To get the fullest stretch, the muscle must be warm. Therefore, if the athlete is stretching in the winter, he should wear long pants or a sweat suit while stretching. In warm weather, shorts are appropriate. Care should be taken to make sure that the muscles do not become cold and stiff during the game or practice session; the athlete should always be trying to stay loose.

In all of these stretches where you are trying to make a maximum effort or bend, try to hold the point of full extension between 5 and 15 seconds.

STANDING STRETCHES

Exercises: Always start with the upper body and proceed downward.

Rotary Arm Swing

Make large circles with the arms so that they completely surround the head and cause a 360 degree rotation of the shoulder joint. This should be performed forward and backward. Make the largest circles you can in each direction. Do at least 8 circles forward and backward. This stretches the deltoids (the top of the shoulders), the pectoralis major (the chest), the trapezius (the shoulders), and the latissimus dorsi (the lats).

Arm Crosses

Vigorously cross the arms in front of the body at about shoulder height. The crossing should be both forward and backward. Be sure to throw the arms across the chest as vigorously as possible to assure the maximum stretch.

Perform at least 8 crosses. This stretches the pectoralis major (chest muscles) and the triceps (back of the arms).

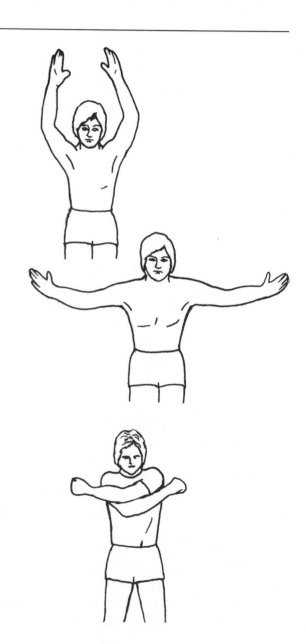

Arm Thrusts (Up and Back)

Throw the arms up and back over the tops of the shoulders as vigorously as possible.

Perform 8 thrusts up and back. This stretches the external obliques (sides of the stomach) and the pectoralis major (chest).

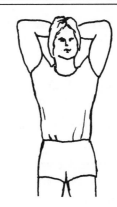

Arm Thrust (Across)

Throw the arms across the body as if elbowing an individual directly behind and punching someone in front. This should be done with enough force so that the breath is exchanged on each turn. An excellent exercise for limbering the back and spine, as well as the shoulders and neck.

Do at least 8 thrusts to each side. This exercise keeps the spine limber and stretches the abdominal muscles.

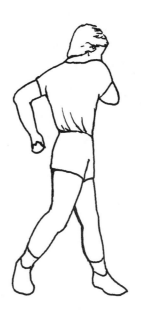
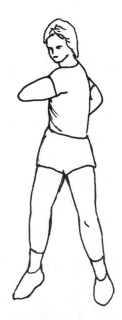

Neck Rotation (Four Way)

Rotate the neck clockwise and then counterclockwise in large smooth circles, then straight forward and backward, and finally from side to side. This is to be followed immediately by shoulder shrugging forward and backward.

Do this at least 8 times in each direction. This exercise keeps the top of the spine limber, relaxes the nerves, and keeps the neck flexible.

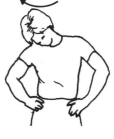
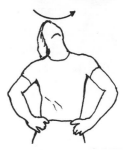
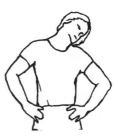
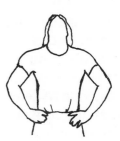

Preparation for Lower Body Stretching

Lean the upper torso over gently and let the leg muscles become used to the weight of the body for 30 seconds. In all of these stretching exercises smoothness should be emphasized; bouncing or jerking to achieve a position should be avoided as much as possible.

Note: As you get older or if it is very cold, the importance of this preliminary stretch becomes obvious. You must let the large leg muscles get a little loosened before you try to stretch them. You can do this exercise sitting down in the V-stretch form. I suggest that you do this exercise about 30 seconds in season; and if you have not stretched for a while, do it two to five minutes, preferably on the floor. Just relax and let the body weight gradually stretch the muscles.

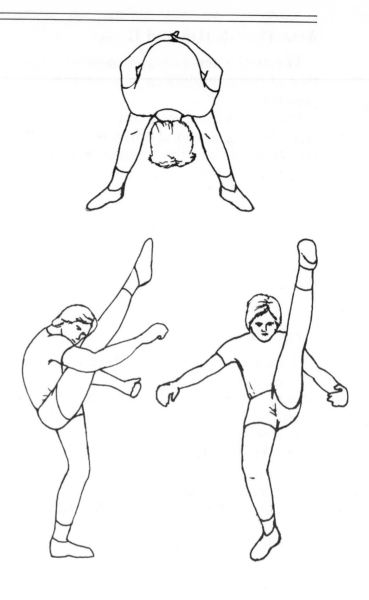

Stiff-Legged Swings

As powerfully as possible, swing the stiff leg straight up and into the chest. Alternate legs after 10 swings. As much effort as possible should be used to keep the other foot firmly on the ground.

This stretches the hamstring and groin muscles of the leg.

Stiff-Legged Circles

Swing the stiff leg up to the chest as before, but this time make a large circle toward the outside at the top of the arch.

This provides a greater stretch for the inner leg muscles. Perform 10 times with each leg.

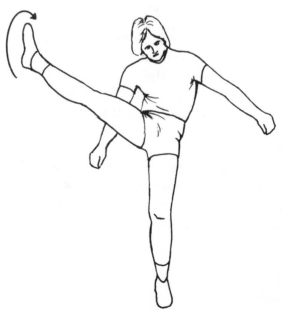

Bent Torso Pulls

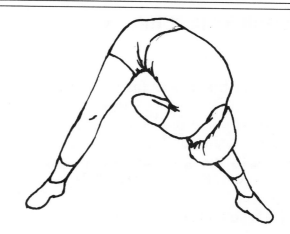

With feet three to four feet apart, lean over as far as possible to try to pull the upper body down to one leg until the chest touches the leg. Turn the waist into the direction of the leg to which you are stretching and try to touch the chest on the thigh. You can pull your body down with your arms by grabbing the leg.

Alternate legs. Do 8 times to each leg, holding for 5 to 15 seconds on the fullest extension. This stretches the calves, the hamstrings, and the groin muscles of the legs. It also supplies back and spine flexibility.

Accentuated Elbow Stretch

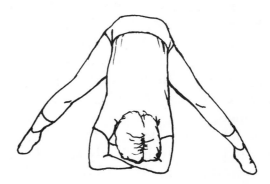

With the legs three to four feet apart, try to touch the elbows to the ground. Try not to bounce but stretch yourself gradually down until you reach the floor. Hold the position for 5 to 15 seconds.

This gives the fullest stretch for the back, the thighs, and the calves.

Groin Stretch

Squat down as far as possible until the tension is felt in the groin area. Now gently rock from side to side, extending first one leg then the other. Then drop to the floor with the arms held straight out. This not only stretches the groin but strengthens it as well.

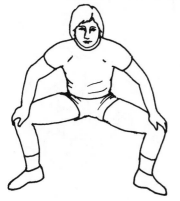
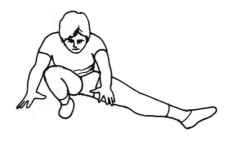
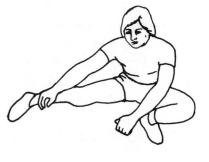

FLOOR STRETCHES

V-Stretch

Spread the legs as far apart as possible, then turn the upper torso into the direction of the leg to which you will stretch. Try to pull the chest down to the leg by using the arms to pull the body down. Hold the stretch for 5 to 15 seconds.

Do 8 stretches to each leg.

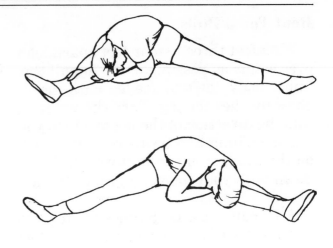

W-Stretch

Keep the legs spread as wide as possible. Throw the arms out and try to touch the toes. At the same time try to touch the floor with your head.

This is a very difficult stretch and requires a lot of back, groin, and hamstring flexibility. It serves as a good test to see if the student is truly stretched.

Do not bounce down to the ground. Let the body weight slowly stretch you down to the ground. Hold this position for 5 to 15 seconds. Do the stretch 8 times.

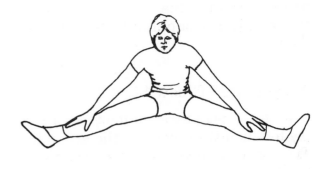

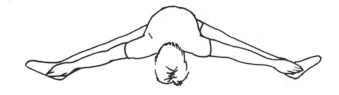

Straight-Legged Stretch

Place the feet and legs together. With the toes pointed, grasp the calves and try to gradually pull the chest down onto the legs until the body rests on top of the legs. (Many athletes cheat on this exercise and only bend the back and touch the face to the legs. This does not provide a full stretch.) Hold yourself down for 5 to 25 seconds, even though you may feel a great deal of discomfort. (This simply means the stretch is working.)

Do the stretch 8 times.

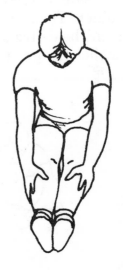

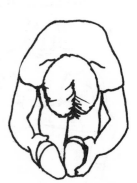

Seated Groin Stretch (Two Parts)

Put the soles of the feet together; gently rock the knees trying to get them to touch the ground on the sides. You can push down with the elbows on the tops of the thighs to help the stretch.

Try to bend over and touch the head to the toes. Do not bounce, but rather pull the body down to the toes. Hold for 5 to 15 seconds.

Do these exercises 8 times.

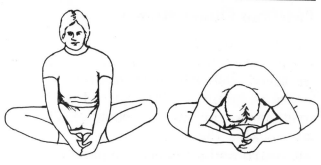

Back Stretching

Roll up on the shoulders, supporting the body with the arms on the ground. Now relax and try to touch the knees to the ground by the sides of the head. Hold this position for 5 to 15 seconds. You only have to do this once. It is very good for keeping the spine limber.

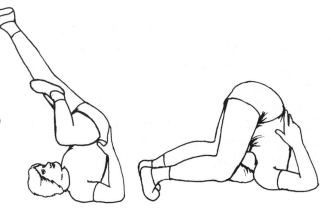

TWO-MAN STRETCHES

Two-Man Standing Stretches

STANDING TO THE FRONT.   One partner grasps the hand of the man stretching and holds onto the leg to be stretched. Now he tries to lift the leg as far up as possible, until the man stretching asks him to stop.

Do this very gradually and easily, 8 times with each leg.

STANDING TO THE SIDE.   This time the partner stands to the side; using a supporting hand lock for balance, he lifts the leg as far up to the side as possible.

Do this slowly and easily, 8 times with each leg.

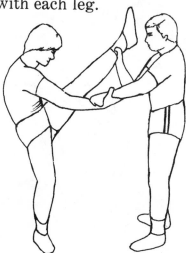

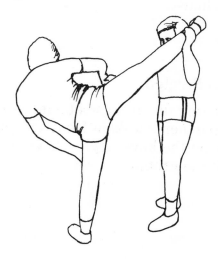

Two-Man Sitting Stretch

SITTING TO THE FRONT.   The partner sits in between the legs of the man to be stretched. Using his own legs for leverage, he pushes the legs of the stretcher as far apart as possible. Then interlocking the grips, he leans backward and stretches the partner down to the ground as far as possible. Important: do this slowly and only stretch the partner as far as he can go without causing too much discomfort. You should do this 8 times and on the last stretch hold the partner down for 5 to 15 seconds.

This is a very good stretching method for athletes who have trouble stretching themselves or seem to be reluctant to do full stretching when exercising.

Straight-Legged Double

Assume the straight-legged stretching stance. The partner stands directly behind and pushes down until the body touches the legs.

The partner should push slowly and only as far as the stretcher can tolerate without too much discomfort.

Do this stretch 8 times and on the last stretch hold the stretcher down for 5 to 15 seconds.

Groin Stretch

Assume the groin stretching position. The partner kneels in front and pushes down on the knees trying to get them to touch the ground.

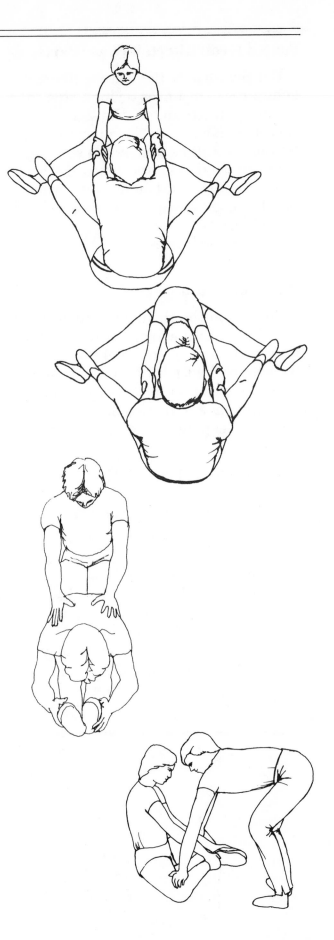

ANKLE ROTATION

Grab the ankle and alternately rotate it forward and backward. Do this rotation at least 8 times in each direction.

Note: It is very important in preventing ankle injuries that the ankle be as flexible as possible; this is a great exercise to increase ankle mobility.

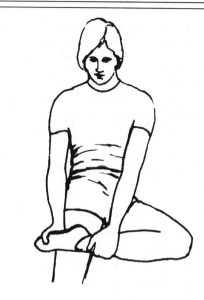

WRIST SHAKING

Shake the wrist vigorously around in circles, then up and down. This helps the wrist to stay flexible and improves coordination.

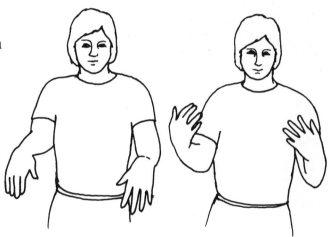

QUESTIONS AND ANSWERS ABOUT STRETCHING

How long should I take each day on my stretches?

Until you are truly stretched you should take about 15 minutes each day to do the full range of stretches found in this program. Remember to take your time and do the stretches slowly and easily so you can get the muscles truly stretched. Evidence of good flexibility is the ability to touch the face to the ground in the V-stretch, the head to the knees in the sitting straight-legged stretch, and the head to the toes in the seated groin stretch. After you have achieved these degrees of flexibility, your program may be shortened to 5 to 7 minutes.

How often should I stretch?

You should stretch every day until you have truly become flexible; thereafter you can stretch three days a week. But if you are practicing every day, you should stretch every day to assure maximum performance and prevent injuries.

What should I wear when stretching?

The warmer the clothes the better, for the muscles always stretch better when they are warm. In the winter you should wear a sweat suit or warm-ups and try to keep the legs and body as warm as possible during practice to keep the maximum flexibility. In the summer you can wear shorts.

How long should I hold each position?

Hold each position at its maximum stretching point for 5 to 15 seconds, breathing very slowly on each stretch and easily when fully stretched. As you become more flexible you will be able to relax more and not experience the pain that is often associated with your early stretching program. Therefore you can hold your stretches longer with more comfort and get better results.

Is any equipment helpful in stretching?

The ballet bar, or stretching bar (a bar several feet long about 3 to 4 feet off the ground) can be very useful in improving your flexibility. You can put your leg on this bar and use your body weight to help your stretches, thereby getting the same results as with the two-man stretches.

How do I keep warm or stretched during the game or a long practice?

When you are on the sidelines, do some simple stretches, such as the arm circles, bend over and grab the legs, touch the elbows to the ground or sit on the ground in the V-stretch or the seated groin stretch. If you find yourself suddenly going into the game, do some quick stiff-legged swings and hand touches to the ground.

CHAPTER 2

Muscle Strengthening

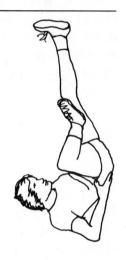

MUSCLE STRENGTHENING WITHOUT WEIGHTS

Often the athlete will not have a weight room available to him, so he must have within his repertoire methods for strengthening his muscles without the use of weights or machines. The muscles will begin to atrophy within 76 hours if they are not stimulated in some fashion that causes them to perform hard work. Floor exercises should be fast, effective, and convenient.

We will work the four major muscle groups of the body using the following sets of floor exercises: (1) pushups for the chest and triceps; (2) sit-ups and leg raises for the abdomen, knees, and groin; (3) jump rope for the arms, legs, and heart.

The body requires approximately 12 minutes of exercise a day in order to stimulate the heart and work the muscles sufficiently to keep them in good shape. The following program takes about 15 minutes and can be done by anyone of any age. It requires no large area, no loud noises, and no particular uniforms.

I suggest that you do these exercises every day that you do not have weights available for training, especially if you are actively engaged in athletics.

Pushups

Four different methods are being used to fully work the chest muscle groups. We shall refer to these as sets.

SET 1. STANDARD PUSHUPS.   Place the hands shoulder width apart, keep on the toes with the back straight and the head straight. Slowly let yourself down until your chest touches the floor, then return to the upright position. Perform 12 of these, then rest 12 seconds until Set 2.

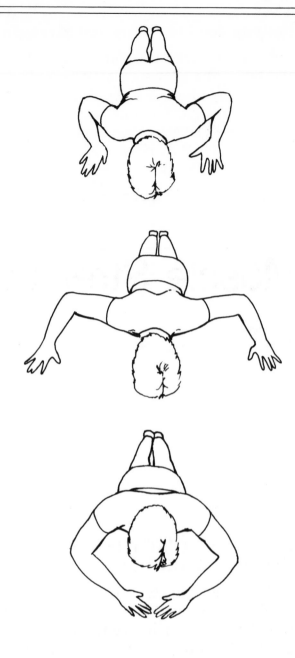

SET 2. WIDE ARM PUSHUPS.   Spread the arms doubly wide. Now go down until your chest touches the floor. Then return to the upright position. Perform 12 of these, rest 12 seconds and proceed to Set 3.

SET 3. HANDS TOGETHER PUSHUPS. Place the hands together to form a small circle at shoulder level. Now slowly let yourself down until your chest touches your hands, then return to the upright position. Perform 12 of these, rest 12 seconds and do Set 4.

SET 4. ARMS OUT PUSHUPS.   Place the arms out in front of the body as far as they can reach. Form a small circle with the hands. Now slowly let yourself down until your head touches the floor. Perform 12 of these, then rest 1 minute until your next floor exercise.

Note: This is the most difficult form of pushup. Do not become discouraged if you have difficulty in doing more than a few. Practice increasing a few each time until you can do 12.

Make it your goal to work up to 25 pushups in each position.

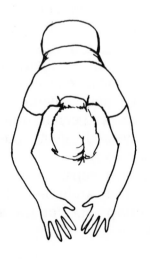

Pushups for Flexibility and Strength

Arch the back up as far as possible and bring the arms in closer to the body, at about chest level. Keeping the arch as much as possible, let the body go through the arms and back up in front of the hands. Hold this position for 5 to 15 seconds and then reverse the procedure.

This pushup is very good for increasing back flexibility and strengthening the spinal column, as well as the arms and chest.

Perform 15 repetitions.

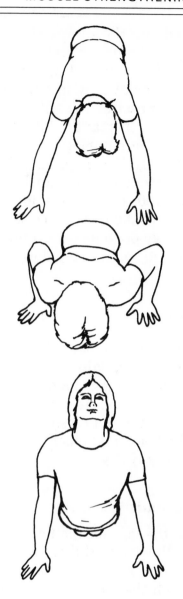

Abdominal Exercises

No other muscle group is as important to the body as the stomach. All movement requires some performance from the stomach muscles. There is no exercise you can do, with or without weights, that in some way does not use the stomach or abdominal muscles.

There are four groups of muscles in the stomach area. Sit-ups work the top two muscle groups; leg raises work the bottom two; side bends work the sides of the stomach or oblique muscles. If you wish to keep a flat stomach as you get older and avoid such things as a "pot gut" or "spare tire" look, then be sure to do many leg raises every day. I suggest that you do up to 100 sit-ups, leg raises, and side bends every day for the rest of your active life.

Sit-ups with a Partner

While letting the partner hold the feet, bend the knees and sit upright. Try to do 100 without stopping.

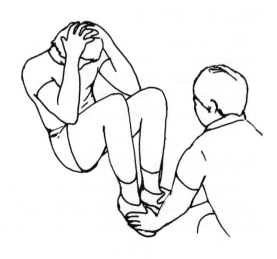

Sit-ups Alone

You may bend your knees, or put your feet under a couch or against the wall if you are doing the sit-ups alone. Try to perform 100 without resting.

Hint: I know 100 sit-ups seems like a lot to you now, but with a few weeks of consistent practice you will be able to do them. It is important to keep a positive mental attitude during this exercise, so try to do only 10 sit-ups at a time, then 10 more, 10 more, etc., until you have achieved 100. But always do 100 before you go on to the next exercise. If you have to stay on your back a few minutes and rest, do so, but stay down until you do 100.

Leg Raises

Lie flat on your back. Place hands under buttocks, palms flat on the floor. Now raise both legs together up to about 60 degrees. (It is not necessary to raise them 180 degrees.) Let them down until the heels just touch the floor. Repeat 100 times.

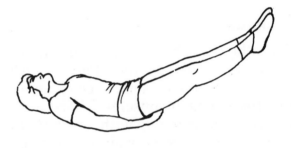

Leg Spreads

Raise the legs off the floor about 6 inches. Now spread them as wide as they can go. Keep the head off the floor and watch the feet. Hold at the maximum spread for 5 seconds, then return. Repeat 25 times.

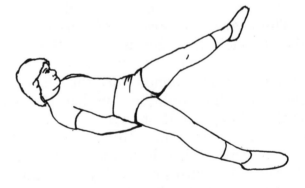

Stomach Beating

Make your hands into fists and hold the legs about 10 inches off the ground with the feet together. Beat as vigorously on the stomach as you can for 15 seconds. Repeat 3 times.

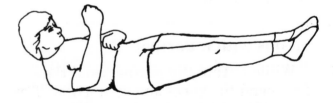

Yoga Stomach Exercise

The purpose of this exercise is to learn to control the stomach muscles. Often we do not have the ability to move our muscle groups as a separate entity, an ability needed when one learns Ki. (See Chapter 5.)

The Stomach Pump

Place the hands on the legs and begin to breathe out slowly. When all the breath is gone, instead of breathing in, feign the inward breath and draw in the stomach muscles very hard as if you were trying to pull the stomach up through the chest. With practice you will be able to suck the stomach in 5 to 8 inches. You can practice by pumping on the stomach as you just start to breathe in.

The Stomach Split

This is a very advanced exercise and requires the utilization of two separate stomach muscle actions. To perform it you must first be able to suck the stomach in as shown in the picture. After the stomach has been sucked in, push very hard on the hands and pull out the middle of the stomach. While using the hands for a push, you suck in on the outer stomach. It is a technique very difficult to describe in words, but not difficult to perform or practice after you have learned the stomach pump.

Jump Rope

Jumping rope is one of the best overall exercises you can do for your muscles and your health. It requires practice to become proficient, but once you have learned to jump, the benefits come quickly and the skill continues to improve very fast. We will concentrate on three exercises: (1) the regular two-legged jump; (2) the one-legged jump; (3) the crossover jump.

The benefits that can be derived from

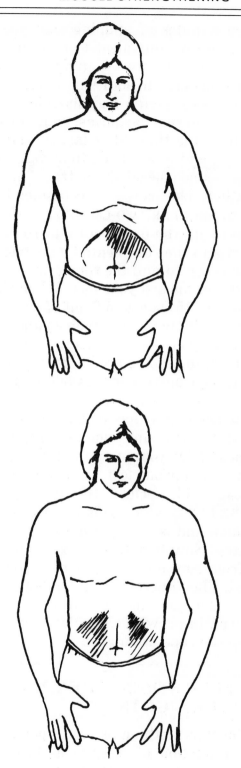

three minutes of jumping continuously are roughly equivalent to nine minutes of jogging because the jumping is done much faster. In addition to using the upper body (arms and shoulders), you get a vigorous cardiovascular workout at the same time. It is faster, more effective, and easier to do than jogging; it requires no special shoes, track, or good weather. That is why I recommend it.

THE REGULAR TWO-LEGGED JUMP. Stand with the feet about 6 to 10 inches apart and the rope behind your back. Now begin to pull the rope over your head and toward your feet. When the rope gets 15 inches in front of your feet, jump up (only about 8 inches) and continue your swing. This takes some practice to become proficient, but do not get discouraged. Perform 300 jumps.

THE ONE-LEGGED JUMP. Stand in the same position as for the two-legged jump, but this time when the rope comes under you, jump up and come down on only one foot. Do about 5 jumps on each foot. Perform 100 jumps.

THE CROSSOVER. This is very hard to explain and is mostly a matter of timing. Simply put, you cross your arms in front as the rope comes over your head. Then uncross them while the rope is in back. Do this 100 times, alternating it with a regular jump to keep the rope untangled.

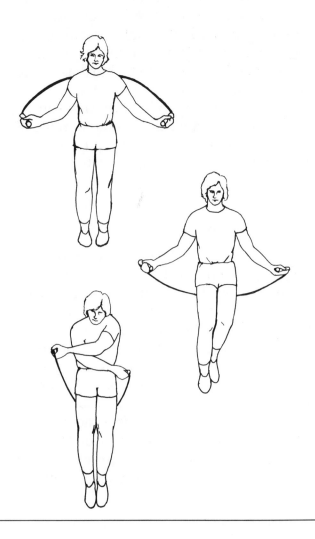

MUSCLE STRENGTHENING WITH WEIGHTS

Perhaps nothing is as important in the reduction of injuries as is muscle tone and muscular strength. However, the importance of the muscles has been overemphasized by many coaches and trainers who regard increasing muscle strength as a cure-all for all problems related to injuries and performance. It is also very important to know how to fall, to be flexible, to utilize balance points, and to practice concentration techniques in order to perform at 100 percent efficiency. I train with weights three days a week and am a firm believer in all forms of weight training. I do not recommend any specific machine or company as the best. They all have points in which they excel, and all have

A WORK OUT CARD FOR THE HIGH SCHOOL ATHLETE:

MEASUREMENTS	0	1 MO.	2 MO.	GOAL
NECK				
SHOULDERS				
ARMS				
CHEST				
WAIST				
HIPS				
THIGH				
CALF				

BRING THIS PROGRAM TO THE GYM MGR OR TO THE INSTRUCTOR ONCE EACH WEEK FOR YOUR PROGRESSION CHECK AND ADJUSTMENT

THIS CARD MUST BE INITIALED BY THE MGR. OR INSTRUCTOR EACH WEEK.
YOUR PROGRESS CHECK AND ADJUSTMENT DAY IS _____

WEEK	1	2	3	4	5	6	7	8	9	10
DATE										
INITIAL										

BUDDY NAMES

NAME	C	J	NAME	C	J

INITIAL   NAME   CARD NO.   SCHEDULE   DATE

Health Progress Chart

EXERCISE:	MUSCLE GROUP	EQUIPMENT USED	SETS	REPS.	INCREASE FOR EACH WEEK									
					1	2	3	4	5	6	7	8	9	10
Leg Extension	Knees	Leg. Mach.	4	6										
Squats	Thighs	Oly. Bar	4	6										
Bench Press	Pects.	Bench	4	6										
Dips	Pects.	Dip Bar	4	6										
Shoulder Press	Delts.	Oly. Bar	4	6										
Shoulder Shrugs	Traps.	Oly. Bar	4	6										
Pull Ups	Lats.	Pull Up Bar	4	6										
Lat. Machine Pull	Lats.	Lat. Mach.	4	6										
Arm Curls	Biceps	Curl Bar	4	6										
Tricep Pushdown	Tricep	Lat. Mach.	4	6										
Sit Ups	Abd.	Incline	4	6										
Leg Ups	Lwr abs.	Incline	4	6										
Side Bends	Abds.	Floor	4	6										
Jump Rope	All	Rope	1	300										

MGR. _____

shortcomings. Weight training will produce excellent results if it is done regularly, if it is supervised, and if it is combined with a proper diet.

A Workout Program to Gain Strength

It does not matter what area of the body you wish to gain your strength in. This formula is utilized by the Russian Olympic weight lifting team and will serve as an outline for the best way to increase strength. Always warm up the body before these exercises (ride a bike, jump rope, etc.).

Warm up with 50 percent of your maximum lift. Do 8 to 10 repetitions, rest 1 minute. Lift 80 percent of your maximum 6 times, rest 1 minute. Lift 90 percent of your maximum 4 times, rest 1 minute. Lift 95 percent of your maximum 2 times, rest until mind is set, not more than 3 minutes. Lift maximum 1 time.

Come down to 90 percent of maximum 2 times, rest 1 minute. Come down to 80 percent of maximum 4 times, rest 1 minute. Come down to 70 percent of maximum 6 times, rest 1 minute. Then do not lift anymore on that exercise that day. You may feel like doing some more sets, but do not do them. This keeps you psyched up and ready. Do not try to lift your maximum more than once every 7 to 12 days.

QUESTIONS AND ANSWERS ABOUT MUSCLE STRENGTHENING

How often should I exercise?

It is recommended that you give the muscle groups rest at least 48 hours but not more than 76 between exercise periods. That gives the muscles time to recover adequately without fatigue. Therefore if you are doing a full body exercise program, do not exercise more than three days a week, or every other day. If you are doing a six-day workout, then work two muscle groups a day (for example, one day concentrate on the arms and chest, one day the legs and lats, one day the shoulders and back, etc.).

What is the best exercise?

There is no one best exercise for everybody. Everyone has his weak points and strong ones. Find your weak ones and work them harder until you make them as strong as your best ones. If you have no way to use weights and are too lazy to do my full floor program, then jump rope and do sit-ups and leg raises every day.

What poundage of weights should I use?

Use a weight that is sufficiently heavy so that by the time of your fourth set you are just barely able to complete the sixth repetition. It is better to have to go down on the last set than to breeze through it. It is not good to start out so heavy that you do not complete any set.

What about protein and diet?

If you want to gain muscle very quickly, I suggest you eat a lot of extra protein (which is what muscles are made of). You can do that by eating a lot of meat, or by taking one of the many brands of protein powder or liquid on the market today. Be careful that you do not gain weight too fast and get fat instead of muscle. I do not recommend that you try to gain more than 5 pounds a month if you want it to be all muscle.

CHAPTER 3

Beginning Mind Control

Mind control is the conscious ability to concentrate the mind toward a specific goal or on a specific muscle, with such determination and persistence that nothing will stop you or break your concentration. It is not a magical power that will make you superman, able to move objects, or change your life or personality. It is your will exercising itself on your conscious and subconscious mind to will it or make it perform and concentrate on one specific object or idea.

The purposes of these exercises are to begin to exert the will on the mind and to begin to let the mind become more powerful in its ability to concentrate. When you are able to truly concentrate the power of the mind on the muscles of your body, the results can be spectacular. They may serve as reinforcement to

you of the power of the mind, and also may convince your muscles of the power the mind has over them. After all, your mind really controls your muscles. The mind tells the muscles what to do and when to do it. The muscles have no control over the mind; the mind is not limited by the muscles and their strength or lack of strength. The mind is potentially the most powerful weapon or force you have. What you want to do now is train it to develop this power within it.

We have all heard the stories of the woman who lifted the car off her son who was trapped under it, or of people who did other apparently superhuman things in time of great stress or excitement. They certainly did not become stronger in a flash and then lose it in the same flash. They only became more determined, more resolved, and concentrated on a job that had to be done immediately. A matter of life and death—no other thought in the mind except the action to perform. After the deed was done they were just as amazed as you or I that they were able to do it. The mind has the potential to move mountains, whether by force or by the invention of machines to blow the mountain up. Just as you give your mind exercises to make it smarter, you can give it exercises to make it stronger. For example, you give it math problems to learn to think abstractly; give it concentration feats (or Ki exercises) to teach it to grow more powerful.

In these exercises you are experiencing only positive reinforcement; you will not get hurt and you will not (if done according to instruction) ever experience a negative result. For example, when you are learning to have an unbendable wrist, you will never let your instructor bend your wrist. You stop him before he is able to. So the mind becomes programmed to expect only positive results and gradually becomes determined to have only Positive Results.

The student should practice the following techniques until he has mastered them. At that time he will have begun to exhibit some sort of conscious control over his mind without losing or breaking his concentration; he will have shown an ability to concentrate on one action until he can do it perfectly.

UNBENDABLE ARM

Just as a tree limb cannot be bent and just as water cannot be compressed, the arm is capable of not being bent when the mind directs it so. The first step is to concentrate on the arm and to continue to tell the arm: "This arm cannot be bent." Then place the arm on the shoulder of the partner, who should place both of his arms near the elbow joint and begin to try to bend the arm. The man trying not to have his arm bent must be careful not to roll the arm over and point the elbow up, for this assures that the arm cannot be bent but also that it can be broken. The student should project a mental image of himself walking forward and through the opponent. This should be practiced a little each day until the time that the arm cannot be bent by the partner. Both arms should be used. The ability to have unbendable arms can be very valuable in stiff arming an opponent in football and in throwing objects.

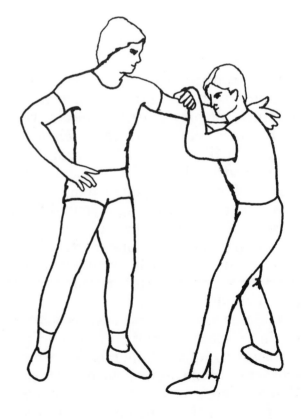

Steps in the "Unbendable Arm"

1. Stand with the feet shoulder width apart and place your arm on the partner's shoulder.

2. Pull him toward you so that you do not have to pull your arm out of its socket, or extend it out, to reach him.

3. Affirm to yourself "this arm cannot be bent."

4. Let your partner begin to pull down on the arm, slowly but with increasing pressure as he pulls.

5. Slowly let your breath out, and let the arm bend slightly with his pulling down efforts.

6. Now asserting your mind, your muscles, and your breath, straighten the arm up and do not allow it to bend again.

7. Repeat with each arm daily until mastered.

8. When partner is trying to bend your arm, if you feel it bending *stop him* and start over. Caution: Do not roll the elbow up; this will break the arm. Do not let the partner jerk hard on the arm; let him pull slowly and steadily.

Results

Increased ability to concentrate; increased muscular control; increased confidence in yourself and your strength and ability; training of the mind to control the muscles. These skills are applicable to many sport situations (stiff arming in football, pushing weights, throwing objects in track and field).

UNBENDABLE WRIST

Using as much mind control and as little muscle as possible the student should attempt to hold his wrist straight and not let it be bent backward by the partner. Exhale the breath during this trial; do not let the wrist be bent while learning. In order to achieve this, when the student feels his wrist about to bend, he should tap his leg or say stop and then begin to concentrate again in another trial. This gives the student only positive reinforcement and will greatly improve his positive mental attitude. He should picture pushing the wrist straight up into the partner's face.

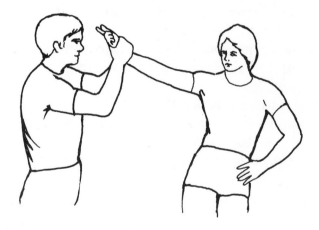

Steps in the "Unbendable Wrist"

1. Stand with the feet shoulder width apart and place your wrist in the partner's hands.

2. Concentrate on the index finger and on the fact that your wrist "cannot be bent."

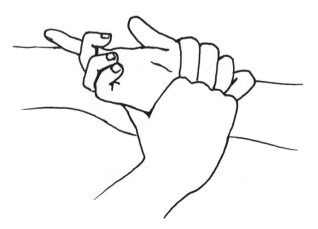

3. Slowly exhale your air, as the partner tries to bend your wrist backward.

4. If you feel the wrist bending, stop the trial and begin a new one.

5. Imagine that you are pushing your wrist up into the sky, or into partner's face.

6. Practice daily until mastered. (This should take from one to four weeks to master.)

Cautions

Do not let the partner bend the wrist on the trials. This can hurt the wrist and give negative reinforcement.

Results

Increased ability to concentrate; increased muscular control; increased confidence in yourself; training of the mind to control the muscles.

INSEPARABLE ARMS

This is a simple matter of leverage, but serves to reinforce a positive mental attitude in the student. With the arms interlocked by the fingers and held at shoulder height, let two partners grab the student on the bicep area, not the forearm, and try to pull (not jerk) the arms apart. Even if as many as four men try, they will not succeed in pulling the arms apart. *Note:* If a football is carried like this, it is impossible to fumble.

This exercise shows how many misconceptions we have about the body. When the arms are placed in this position, they actually are already apart. Note that the shoulders and elbows are fully extended to the sides. The only thing that is together is the fingers, and the partners are not trying to pull the fingers apart—they are trying to separate the arms, which are already apart. So unless they jerk or pull from the front, they cannot pull the arms apart.

This technique does have practical applications. If you wrap your arms around someone you wish to tackle in football, they will not be able to make you let your arms go. You may not tackle them, but at least they will drag you over the goal line and you won't look as bad as if you had let them go.

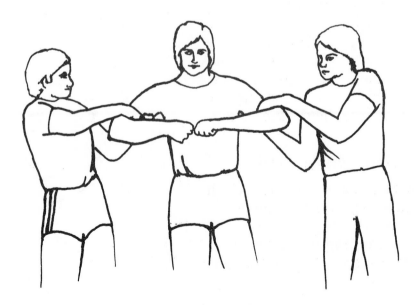

ARM ON HEAD

This exercise also reinforces a positive mental attitude in the student. In addition, it can serve as a maneuver in sports (such as in basketball when the ball is grabbed from the backboard near the head). No matter how strong or powerful the partner, the arm cannot be separated from the top of the head—it is quite easy to follow a downward pull and it is impossible for the partner to pull the arm off upward.

CHAPTER 4

Balance and Leverage Points

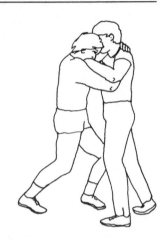

Perhaps no other concept is more misunderstood in America than the benefits that can be derived from the proper use of balance and leverage points. Imagine the human being as a statue. If you did not glue the statue onto the base or stand, it certainly would not stand up. You cannot build something that is six feet tall and weighs 200 pounds and balance it on something 12 inches long and 4 inches wide—or if you could balance it, it would be the easiest thing in the world to knock over with just a touch of the fingers. It is actually the same thing with people. It took you two years to learn to walk; and even today if you hurt or lose a toe, you will limp the rest of your life. Your balance is a very delicate thing; it requires the use of the many organs and senses of the body all at once to stay in equilibrium. You have to have the coordination of the inner ear, the eyes, the brain, the toes, the arms, and the hips to stay upright or to move forward with any grace or without falling.

Any person, no matter how he stands or how he is moving, is off balance in eight positions. Just like the statue that can be pushed over with one hand, he can be pushed over or moved about with the greatest of ease by the proper use of the balance and leverage points. (A child can support a 400 pound refrigerator that has been tipped on its corner if he can just maintain the proper balance.) So size and strength can be effectively overcome by the smallest of persons if they make effective use of balance and leverage points. Balance is essential in an athlete's performance. When properly understood, it can be very valuable as an offensive and defensive tactic.

EIGHT POINTS OF BALANCE

No matter how the student may stand, there are eight points of balance (or lack of balance) when a line is drawn between the feet. These points correspond with points on a clock, with 12 o'clock directly behind and 6 o'clock directly in front of the student. The other points are where 2, 3, 4, 8, 9, and 10 o'clocks would fall. If the position of the feet is not changed, the partner can easily push or pull the student off balance by using one of these points.

It is, therefore, quite possible to push or pull an opponent all over a field by causing him to lose his balance and keeping him off balance.

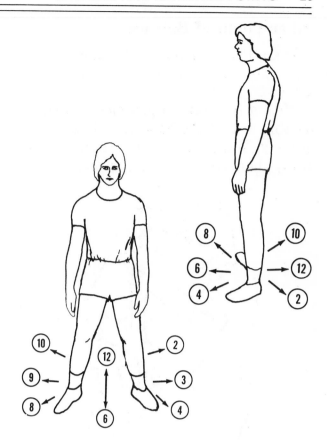

Primary Balance Point

To make effective use of the balance points, one must become very familiar with where these points are at various times and with various feet positions of the partner.

The primary balance point and the one easiest to use is the 12-6 balance point. This point is found by drawing a line straight through the ankles of the partner and then drawing a perpendicular line directly out from the middle of the line between his feet. The partner will then be able, by the slightest use of his arm, to push the partner backward to the 12 or pull him forward to the 6. The partner will not fall over because he will move his feet and keep his balance. If he did not move his feet, he would fall over. In a game this movement is involuntary and can be used to make blocks, tackles, move an opponent, or avoid an attack.

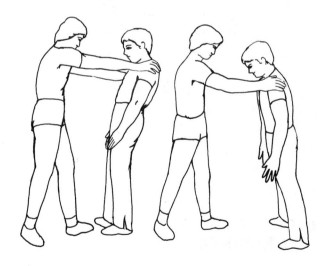

Other Points of Balance

The other six points of balance correspond to the 3, 9, 2, 8, 4, and 10 on a clock.

With a few days of practice you will be able to find the balance points quickly. You should be able to begin to apply them to your sport, with the help of your coach, and by using common sense and trial and error experimentation.

To practice in the most effective manner, the partners should change feet position and try to find the balance points in each of these positions.

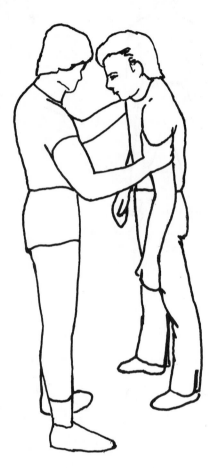

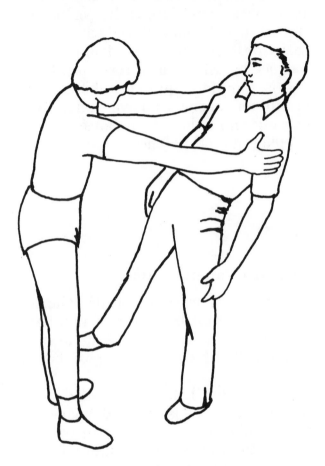

CIRCLING AND NONRESISTANCE

A simple rule to remember is: "if they push, you pull; if they pull, you push." If you begin to use this rule you can stop the biggest of opponents and overcome the strongest of assaults. Force can be applied in only one direction. You cannot push forward and up at the same time, or to the right and left at the same time. The force in its direction of movement has the power. It has no power in the direction it is not moving because it is not there at all.

The three pictures on this page show the push-pull method. Instead of pushing back against the opponent, you should grasp his arms and let him push you backward. Then take a slight step and pull him. Then his strength becomes your strength. Now throw him past you and continue to walk forward.

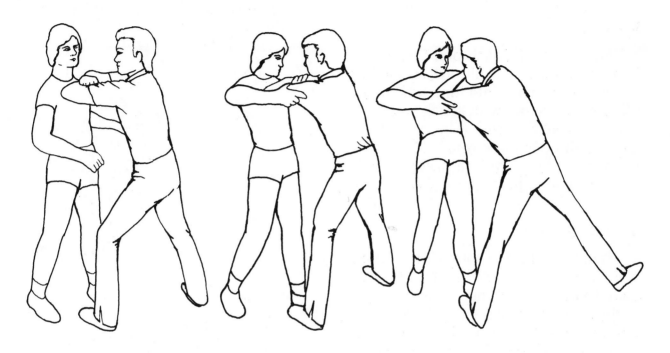

SPECIALIZED TECHNIQUES FOR APPLYING BALANCE AND LEVERAGE TO FOOTBALL SITUATIONS

Blocking

Often when blocking it becomes a matter of who weighs more or is stronger. However, if you will use speed and balance to step between the legs of the opponent, you can effectively counter his size and strength.

As you keep off the line, instead of just pushing your body weight against him, step very far with your lead leg until it is between the legs of the opponent. This utilizes his 6-12 balance points and causes him to fall backward

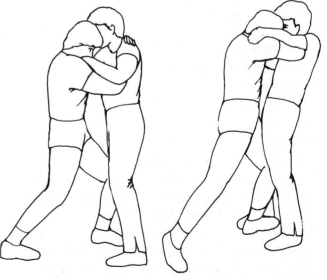

or at least move backward. It takes just a little practice to take the longer step between the man's legs, but once mastered it is very fast and extremely effective.

Rushing

This utilizes the push-pull theory. Instead of letting the blocker smash into you and you smash into him, let him use all of his force to try to knock you backward. Grasp hold of his shoulders and let him push into you; use his momentum to throw him past you as you continue to pursue the play.

Tackling

Often you will find yourself (weighing 175 pounds) in the backfield with a 240-pound fullback rushing toward you. Unless you are really exceptional you will not be able to meet this man head on and tackle him. However, you can use his momentum to your advantage. Instead of trying to stop him by a head-on tackle, just try to use his balance point to pull him directly to the ground, which is already the direction in which his head is pointing.

As you begin to make contact with the ball carrier, simply grasp hold of him and let him continue to run toward and over you.

Now hold tight on him and fall directly onto your back, pulling down sharply with your arms and body weight. He will usually fall down on top of you, especially if you tangle his feet up by placing yours between his as he is running over you. *Remember:* He is trying to run forward and you are not preventing him from running forward. You are simply pushing his forward momentum into the ground and causing him to fall.

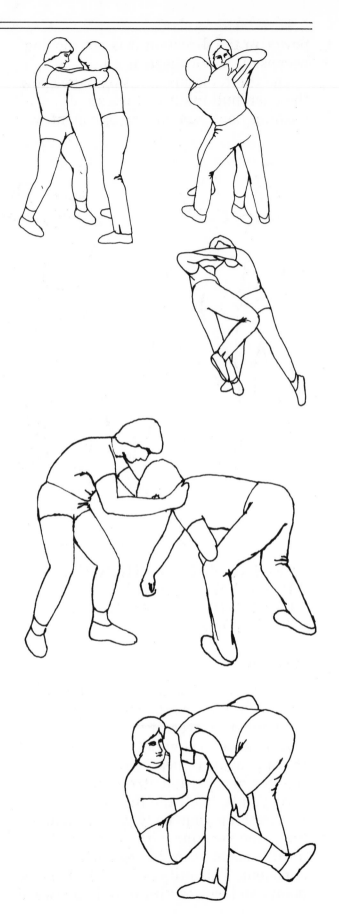

Moving a Player

If you find yourself holding onto a big man and trying to move him to either side with just the strength of your arms, you will often find yourself unable to do it; he shifts his weight just as you try to move him and becomes too heavy for you to move. To overcome this, you must fake a move to the right and then quickly reverse your move directly to the left, utilizing the 3-9 balance point.

Grasp the man at his shoulders and attempt to move him to the right. As he begins to shift his weight to the right to prevent this, immediately snap your movement to the left. If you are quick enough, he will fall to the left and you can continue pursuit.

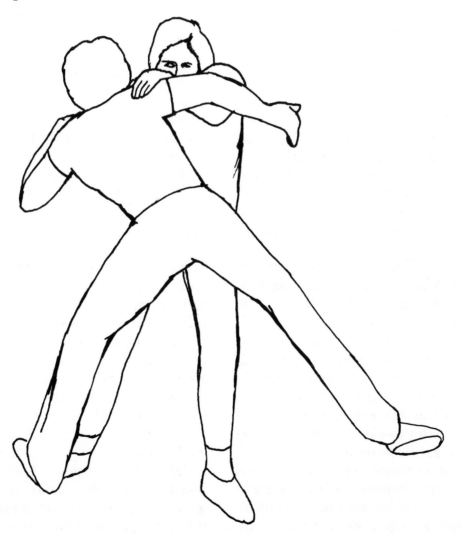

CHAPTER 5

Ki (Muscle, Breath, and Mind Control)

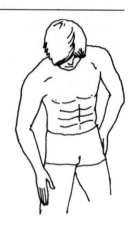

This chapter deals with a concept that is unfamiliar to many Americans, but understood and practiced by most Orientals. The concept of Ki is 3,000 years old and was developed by the Buddhist monks of the Sholan Monastery of China.

Ki is a product of three separate forces. (1) Muscle control—the instantaneous tightening of specific muscles at the moment of impact. (2) Breath control—the movement of the breath, forcibly, at the instant of impact to allow the muscles full contraction, and to strengthen the concentration of the mind. (3) Mind control—the concentration of the mind toward a specified area of the body about to be hit.

When these three forces are joined together, they become a single force called Ki. Ki can be used to prevent an injury from a punch or a blow, to in-crease determination, to give courage, to improve skills, to increase strength, and to develop concentration.

Why does your Ki work? It works because you are using all the powers of your body, not just your muscle, to prevent an injury. Many people think that muscle alone can prevent an injury from a blow. But this is not the case as is illustrated in the two examples that follow. (1) If someone were to hit you hard in the leg, which is all muscle, you would at the least get a bruise—perhaps a charley horse or a muscle injury. That is because the leg is actually too much muscle and as such cannot give any with the blow. It is like a tree covered with snow that finally breaks under the weight of the snow. A smaller, more flexible tree can bend and touch the ground and not break. Your leg has all muscle and no give, so a hard blow breaks the muscle tissue and causes the bruises. (2) It is also possible to make the stomach very strong by the use of sit-ups and leg raises; then if you tighten your stomach muscles you can let someone punch you there. However, take a deep breath of air into your stomach and then let someone hit you there. A very slight blow would cause a significant amount of damage—the air acts like a balloon and explodes or pops in the stomach area causing internal damage. Let us suppose that you can take a punch in the stomach and you have let most of your air out. But before you are ready for the punch, someone comes up and asks you a question, momentarily distracting you, and you are hit. Needless to say, you could be very seriously injured because your mind was not prepared for the blow.

So you can see it takes all three techniques to protect the body from injury. First, you must have adequate muscle and muscle control so that you can tighten and contract the muscles at the point of the impact of the blow. Secondly, you must have some breath control and be breathing out, or moving your breath away from the area getting hit. Finally, you must have your mind controlled and aware that you are getting hit so you can concentrate the muscles and breath simultaneously at the point of impact.

With these three factors working for you, your Ki is said to be "flowing" and you are able to resist blows that would cripple untrained people. You have been able, by practice and the use of positive reinforcement and progressive training, to apply your muscle, breath, and mind to such states that you can focus them simultaneously and instantaneously on the area of impact when you see a blow about to occur.

We have studied exercises that strengthen the muscles (see Chapter 2) and those that help the mind to concentrate (see Chapter 3). Now we will begin to do exercises to strengthen breath control.

The first step in controlling the breath is to become aware of it as a force, and to use it to store power (or concentration effort) in the lower body. *Note:* The center of gravity is located about two inches below the navel and serves as a focus point for the mind when developing control of the breath and understanding of Ki.

BREATHING EXERCISES

Stomach Breathing

The purpose of this exercise is to focus the attention of the mind on the center of gravity, or lower consciousness of the body, and to store your Ki (or concentration power) in your body. What you should be thinking when you are doing this exercise is that you are storing a power in your body and this power will be used to prevent your injuries. While you are practicing the breathing, keep thinking that you are storing a power in your body.

Procedure: Stand with the feet shoulder width apart, with the arms by the sides and the hands closed into fists. Keep the mouth shut and breathe through the nose. Keep the back straight and the neck and heart in a straight line. Begin to breathe in slowly, but instead of filling your chest with air, breathe into the stomach, filling it with air. Hold it a few seconds and begin to breathe out slowly, pulling in on the stomach gently as you breathe out. Hold it a few seconds and repeat the exercise. Do this exercise for two minutes, all the time concentrating on the lower stomach area and thinking you are storing a power in your lower body. *Note:* If you get restless and begin to lose your concentration, stop the exercise. This exercise only works when you believe and concentrate on the fact that you are storing a power and when you keep the mind concentrated on your breathing. You are doing this exercise both to control your breath and to practice mind focus or concentration. Do this every day for at least three months, and then at least twice a week after you have developed your Ki sufficiently to receive very hard blows without injury.

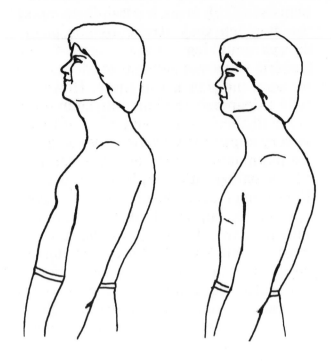

Isotonic Breathing

The purpose of this exercise is to begin to learn how to get all of the air out of the body, especially the stomach area, by the concentration of the mind and the tightening of the muscles to help to squeeze the air out. This is a five part exercise and should be performed immediately after the stomach breathing exercise. Procedure:

1. Place the feet together, and keep the back straight. Slowly begin to raise the arms straight up above the head to a full extension. While raising the arms straight up, begin to let the air out of the stomach and chest; as you get to the top, begin to tighten the muscles of the entire body to squeeze every last drop of air out of the stomach and the chest. Hold this position for three seconds; concentrate on tightening every muscle

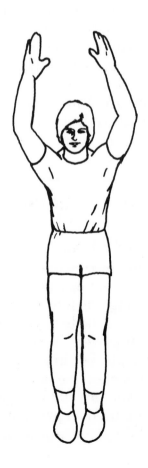

of the body to help squeeze the air out.

2. Bring the arms back to the level of the shoulders and slowly begin to push the arms out straight to the sides. While pushing the arms out to the sides, continue to tighten every muscle of the body to get every ounce of air out of the body. Hold your full extension for three seconds; again, really concentrate on getting all the air out of the body and on the tightening of all muscles of the body.

3. Slowly bring the arms back to the level of the shoulders. Begin to push them out straight ahead of the body. While pushing the arms straight ahead concentrate to tighten all the muscles and to squeeze all the air out of the body. Hold your full extension straight ahead for three seconds. Now slowly return the arms to the shoulders.

4. Slowly push the arms straight down in front of the body. Concentrate all the muscles to squeeze the air out. Hold your full downward extension for three seconds and then slowly bring the arms up to the chest.

5. Open the legs, tighten the fists, and lean over slightly. Concentrate on tightening all the muscles of the stomach as hard as you can. Try to crunch down the stomach muscles and squeeze the stomach muscles together (like an accordion). Do this about 15 seconds until you really begin to feel all the muscles of the stomach tightening.

This exercise is excellent for learning to get the air out of the body, especially out of the stomach area. It helps practice mind control and concentration techniques plus strengthens the muscles through isometric contraction.

Perform this exercise daily for at least three months until you can let someone hit you very hard in the solar plexus area and the ribs. Then you may practice it two to three times a week.

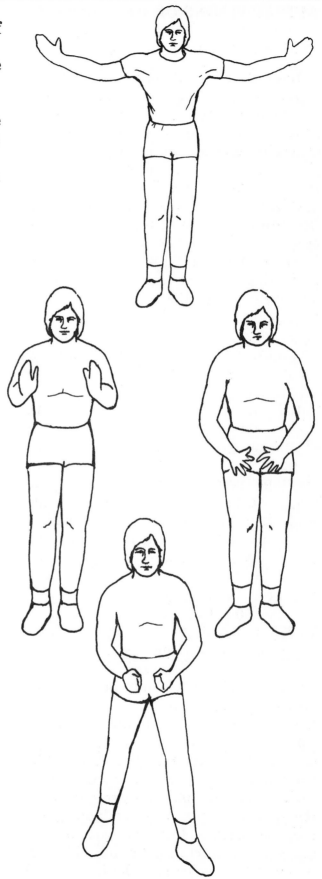

APPLICATIONS OF KI

Taking a Punch in the Stomach

You are now ready to apply your concept of Ki by learning to take a punch in the stomach. We have already begun to practice the three aspects that are necessary to develop our Ki. We are doing sit-ups, leg raises, and muscle conditioning exercises to strengthen the muscles and learn to control them. We are doing breathing exercises that help us move our breath from various areas of our body that may be hit. We have practiced beginning mind control to learn to focus and concentrate the mind on one specific point, or to one area of the body. Now we will use all three at once and begin to see how easy it is to let someone hit us in the stomach without receiving an injury or even a bruise.

1. Stand with the feet shoulder width apart. Concentrate the mind on the fact "I am going to get hit in the stomach." Repeat this thought over and over, at the same time saying to yourself "I am not going to get hurt; I cannot be hurt by a hit in the stomach." Your mind has fantastic power when it is concentrated in this way. If it believes firmly that you are going to get hit in the stomach, it will prepare all the muscles of the body for the blow and will begin to concentrate the breath as it has learned from the breath-controlling exercises. Next, when the mind tells your body "I am not going to get hurt," your body has no choice but to react as if it were not going to get hurt. Your muscles cannot think; your breath cannot think. They do not know if the person punching you can hurt you or not. Your mind must make that decision. You are conditioning your mind now by affirming to yourself the positive fact that you are not going to get hurt. Your mind will coordinate the muscles and the breath and

prepare the body for the blow; the combination of the three factors will assure that you do not receive an injury.

Note: You will never get hurt when practicing. First of all, you will not be experiencing negative reinforcement, because you will be using a partner who will use his fingertips for the first punch in the stomach and will not hit you any harder until you are ready for a harder punch. Each time you train, your confidence will be built up and your Ki will become stronger because of practice. By the time you are ready to let someone hit you very hard, your mind is ready, your breath is ready, and your muscles are ready.

2. Step forward with either foot, and let half of the air out of the stomach area. (Do not let all of the air out because the partner may wait until you breathe in and then hit you. This can do damage.) Continue to really concentrate on the two important facts. "I am going to get hit," and "I will not get hurt."

3. When you are firmly convinced that you are ready to take the punch and that you will not be hurt, nod your head and the partner will lightly hit you in the stomach. Keep your eyes open, and as you see the punch coming, quickly begin to tighten all the stomach muscles and all the other muscles of the body. At the same time exhale all your air as forcefully as you can and make a noise when doing so. (You cannot let all your air out forcefully unless you are making a noise.) Some students are shy or reserved and do not want to make a loud noise. Let me assure you that the louder the noise, the more power you are bringing into your stomach area—power of concentration, muscle control, and breath.

4. When the punch hits your stomach, yell as loud as you can; tighten all the muscles and then keep the body and breath ready in case another punch is to follow. (Sometimes in a game you will get hit twice.) After you are certain no more punches are coming, step back and smile, reconfirming to yourself that you were not hurt and you won't ever be hurt by these exercises. (This is to practice your positive conditioning.) Do not let the partner hit you several times in the beginning, unless you concentrate completely the mind each time as you did to take the first punch.

5. Each time you practice, you should increase the power of the punches that the partner is using. In a very short time you will be able to let him hit you as hard as he can without your receiving any injury or bruise.

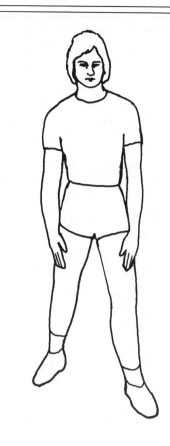

REVIEW. First concentrate the mind on two facts: "I am going to get hit in the stomach" and "I am not going to get hurt."

After you have accepted and believed these facts, step forward and let out half of your breath. Continue your concentration and nod your head when you are ready for the partner to hit you.

At the instant of impact let out all your air as forcefully as you can, with a loud noise. Tighten every muscle of your body. Keep believing that it can't hurt you.

As you learn the proper technique for letting all your air out, tightening the muscles, and concentrating the mind, you can receive progressively harder punches. In the beginning, however, it is not necessary or advisable to let yourself be given more than a tap.

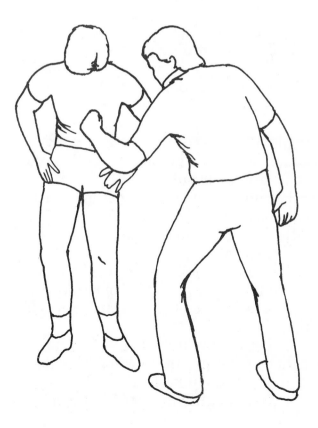

Taking a Punch in the Ribs

You have probably never been told

what you could do to protect the ribs if you were going to get hit there. Fortunately, such protection is available in a form of Ki that can be learned quickly and applied to most game situations.

Remember that when you are getting hit in the ribs you are doing something, even if it is only letting your ribs get broken. Most people do exactly the wrong thing when they feel a hit coming into the ribs. They try to get out of the way. This stretches the rib cage open and lets a lot of air into the chest. We have already seen that air can burst like a balloon, and certainly if you expose your ribs and separate them by leaning away from the blow, you will get them cracked or broken by the hit.

What you should do is rely upon the three factors of your Ki. Let the large muscle groups of the abdominal and the lats cushion and absorb most of the blow; at the same time let the breath be forcefully exhaled to keep the rib cage contracted as fully as possible and use the mind to concentrate your power to the area to make your muscles and breath react properly. If you do these three things, the blow will just bounce off and cause no damage or pain.

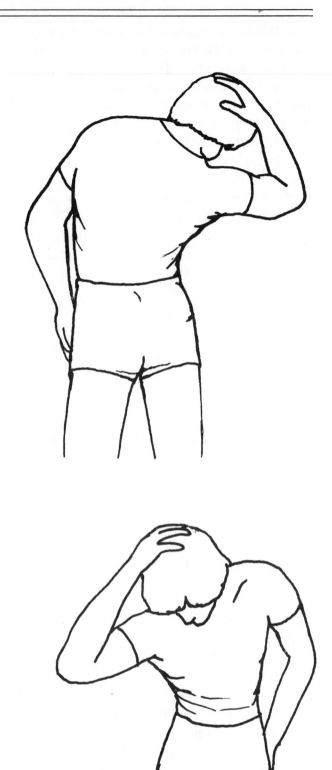

PROCEDURE. When practicing, place the hand on top of the head; in most games when you get hit in the ribs your arms are up or out.

1. Pull the lats muscle out as far as possible. Concentrate the muscles of the latissimus dorsi and make them larger or expanded.

2. Lean the body to the side being hit; try to touch the elbow to your side—this squeezes the ribs together and protects them.

3. Let the breath out forcefully to help you squeeze the ribs together and to contract the muscles.

4. Lean slightly forward in the area

of the blow. This pulls the lats out further to act as a cushion for the blow.

If you are being punched in the floating ribs (the area located at the sides of the abdominal muscles), you must lean forward, crunch down on the stomach and rib cage and into the blow. To get the stomach muscles, which play an important part in this Ki, fully tightened (and the ribs tightened), you must let your breath out at the point of impact.

Note: It is vital that you overemphasize the downward crunching movement of the ribs and the crunch of the stomach muscles.

Taking Strikes in the Neck

One of the most common and dangerous injuries is the neck injury. Many weight lifting machines and numerous neck exercises have been tried to strengthen the neck. But just making the neck stronger is like padding a glass jar and then repeatedly throwing it against the wall. No matter how much padding, someone finally will throw it just right and break the jar. The same is true with the neck. The athlete often just tries to pad it more (or make it stronger) and then keeps butting his head into other people or hitting his head against the wall. Finally one of the blows will be just right and the neck will get injured. It is a much better and safer idea to use your Ki to protect your neck and spine from injury. Remember, we are still relying heavily on the muscles to protect the neck, but now we are adding the protection of the breath and the concentration power of the mind.

PROCEDURE FOR TAKING A STRIKE IN THE FRONT OF THE THROAT OR NECK.

1. Tighten the neck muscles as much as possible.

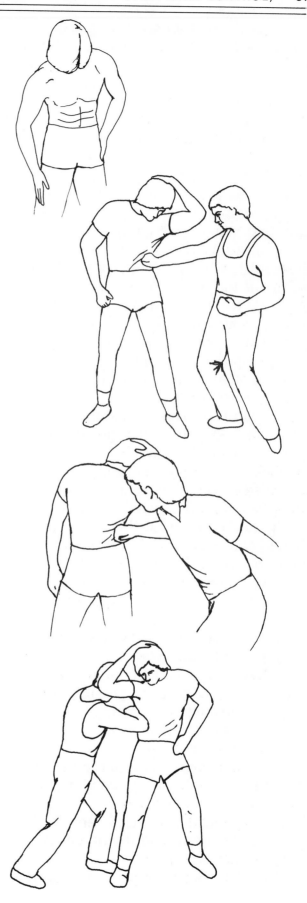

2. Jut the bottom jaw forward so that you have an underbite effect. At the same time pull back on the tongue and make the same muscle contraction you would as when swallowing.

3. Lift the shoulders up, and flex the trap muscles. Tighten the fists to give strength to the trap and shoulder muscles.

4. Focus your mind on the fact that you are going to get struck in the neck and that you are not going to get hurt.

5. Breathe out slowly but extremely forcefully while you wait for the blow; at the instant of impact, really force your air through your neck (but do not make a sound or a noise other than the air escaping from your mouth).

6. Keep the neck muscles and mind concentrated until you are sure no more blows are coming.

You can test to see if you have protected your Adam's apple area or larynx. To do this have your partner try to choke you. If you are doing the exercise correctly, your larynx should float back into the muscle area of your neck and be protected there. Do not bend your neck in such a fashion that your jaw rests on your chest because then you have not protected the neck, but you have exposed the jaw and teeth.

PROCEDURE FOR TAKING A STRIKE IN THE BACK OF THE NECK.

1. Keep the back and spine in a straight line as much as possible. Do not lean forward or backward.

2. Tighten all the muscles surrounding the neck.

3. Exhale your breath forcefully to allow full muscle contraction and to aid your mind concentration.

4. Concentrate the mind very hard on the area being hit and firmly believe you will not be injured.

Notes: The neck can be protected by

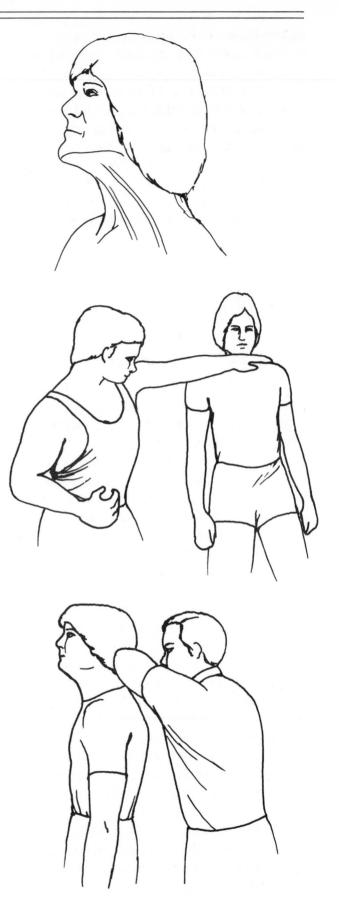

the use of Ki. However, this is a very dangerous area in which to make a mistake while practicing. I do not advise that you ever practice with full power blows to the front or the back of the neck, but rather practice with softer blows so that you can develop your technique and timing; then if you actually were hit there, you could react quickly and correctly.

Even though you do not see the blows coming from behind to the back of the neck, you can be prepared for such blows. Get into the habit of not relaxing the neck muscles and not leaning the neck forward or backward.

PRACTICE SCHEDULE FOR KI

The First Week

DAY ONE.

a. 50 sit-ups, 50 leg raises, 20 side bends

b. stomach breathing 2 minutes

c. isometric stomach breathing, 5-way

d. concentration for at least 30 seconds on "I am going to get hit in the stomach." "I am not going to get hurt."

e. partner just jabs his fingers into solar plexus area. (Be sure to overreact and really tighten the muscles; scream at the instant of impact even though this is a soft blow.)

f. affirmation—affirm to yourself, "That did not hurt, and I cannot get hurt by being punched in the stomach."

DAY TWO.

a. 60 sit-ups, 60 leg raises, 20 side bends

b. stomach breathing 2 minutes

c. isometric stomach breathing, 5-way

d. concentration for at least 30 seconds on "I am going to get hit." "I am not going to get hurt."

e. partner hits you in the stomach with ¼ of his full power. (Be sure to overreact to the punch and greatly tighten the stomach muscles; forcefully exhale the air and scream at the point of impact.)

f. affirmation—"That did not hurt, and I cannot get hurt by being punched in the stomach."

DAY THREE.

a. 70 sit-ups, 70 leg raises, 20 side bends

b. stomach breathing 2 minutes

c. isometric stomach breathing, 5-way

d. concentration for at least 30 seconds (See above concentration thoughts.)

e. partner hits you in the stomach with ⅓ his power. (Be sure to be overready for his punch. In other words be ready for a punch twice as hard as he will give.)

f. affirmation (See above affirmations.)

DAY FOUR.

a. 80 sit-ups, 80 leg raises, 20 side bends

b. stomach breathing 2 minutes

c. isometric stomach breathing, 5-way

d. concentration for 30 seconds

e. partner hits you in the stomach with ½ his power

f. affirmations

DAY FIVE.

a. 90 sit-ups, 90 leg raises, 20 side bends

b. stomach breathing 2 minutes

c. isometric stomach breathing, 5-way

d. concentration for 30 seconds

e. partner hits you in stomach with ⅔ his power

f. affirmations

DAY SIX.

a. 100 sit-ups, 100 leg raises, 20 side bends

b. stomach breathing 2 minutes

c. isometric stomach breathing, 5-way

d. concentration for as long as you need to take a full power punch. Not more than a minute should be needed.

e. partner hits you as hard as he can in the stomach

f. affirmations and congratulations by partner and coach

REST SUNDAY.

Subsequent Weeks

The second week continue to do 100 sit-ups, 100 leg raises, and 20 side bends a day, plus 2 minutes of stomach breathing, and 5-way isometric stomach breathing. Try to lessen the amount of time you need to concentrate, and begin to practice your rib Ki in the same gradual manner you did the stomach Ki. By the end of the week you should be able to take a full-power punch in the stomach and a full-power strike in the ribs.

The third week continue to do 100 sit-ups, 100 leg raises, and 20 side bends a day, plus 2 minutes stomach breathing, and 5-way isometric stomach breathing. Also, increase your concentration ability, take punches in stomach and ribs, and begin to practice techniques for neck Ki (but do not practice taking hard strikes in the neck *ever*, just practice the technique).

Continue to practice your Ki vigorously and religiously every day you can until you have developed the techniques so that you are able to let someone punch you either in the ribs or the stomach without more than a split second notice, and until you can take several strikes in a row to different areas of your body. As your mind gets stronger and your breath and muscle control become sufficient so that you are absolutely assured of their immediate and full cooperation when you practice your Ki, your Ki will continue to get better.

Ki will work. Ki does work. Ki can be developed by anyone who believes in himself and the power of his mind—his ability not to get hurt no matter how big the person hitting him—and who is willing to work the following program: 100 sit-ups, 100 leg raises, and 20 side bends daily; a regular muscle strengthening program; 2 minutes of stomach breathing every day for at least a month; isometric stomach breathing 5-way; beginning mind control exercises and meditation techniques (see Chapter 11); progressive-positive training with a proper partner.

QUESTIONS AND ANSWERS ON KI

What if you don't see the blow coming?

Nine out of ten times you do see the blow coming because it is illegal in most sports to hit the man from behind. Because you see the blow coming you will be able to react in time. Get in the habit of always being ready when on the field or playing. Don't let your guard down.

Keep the muscles tense but not tight. Keep the breath under control. Do not get lazy and start breathing into the stomach; keep the mind concentrated and prepared for a blow at any time. Remember the play is not over until you are in the huddle, the referee has the ball, or the final gun has blown. I guess the best motto is to "Stay Prepared."

How do I practice without getting hurt?

Practice in progressive steps using only positive reinforcement. Start out with a tap, and only build up the power of the hits a little at a time as your technique progresses and your mind and body become stronger and more confident. Always use a partner who wants to help you learn—not one who wants to hurt you.

How often should I practice my Ki?

You should do your breathing exercises every day, your sit-ups every day, your muscle training three times a week, your meditation and beginning mind control exercises every day for at least three months. By then you will have learned all the techniques well enough to take almost any blow without receiving an injury. Then you may practice these exercises three times a week. Remember that your Ki is as much technique as it is mind control. You must practice your technique by letting people hit you. If you have not let anyone hit you for four weeks, your technique will not be as sharp, therefore your Ki will not be as good. It is just like any sport—you must practice specific techniques quite often to stay in top condition.

When should I not practice?

Do not try to do Ki when you have been drinking (alcohol deludes one into thinking he has more power than he really has). Never do Ki when on drugs, not after eating (wait at least an hour), not just as you wake up (wait until you are fully awake and your mind is very clear). Also if you ever feel like you don't want to get hit, or just don't have any Ki that day, then you are right and you should not practice your Ki. You must wait until your mind is ready to do Ki correctly.

How do I do all these things in a game situation?

You should have the muscle strength from your muscle training, and you can practice your breathing exercises before the game. Use the time you have in the huddle or before the ball is snapped or when you are on the sidelines to keep the mind concentration at a top level.

CHAPTER 6

Removal of Pain

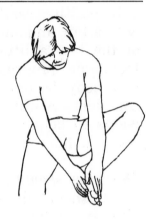

Pain is a defense mechanism used by the body to warn it that an injury is occurring, or has occurred, and to keep it aware of the injured area in order to avoid reinjuring it. Pain is not caused by the injury but is caused by the nerves reacting to the injury. The science of acupuncture and acupressure has developed techniques to stop the nerves from transmitting pain to the brain, thereby stopping the brain from feeling the sensation of pain. Pain must be interpreted by and felt in the brain.

Even though it seems as though the injury is being felt in the area of the damage, actually the pain is being sent to the brain via the nerves, translated and interpreted in the brain, and sent back to the affected area. A cycle is thus formed with the nerves and the brain,

not with the injury and the brain. It is not necessary to experience pain unless the pain is being experienced by the actual injury.

Drugs have been developed to stop pain from being interpreted in the brain. Aspirin is the most popular of such drugs. Some pain-relieving drugs are so strong that surgery can be performed without any pain being experienced during the operation.

There are techniques for avoiding the sensation of pain or preventing and removing the pain syndrome. These techniques are not new and have been used in the Orient for thousands of years. They may have been used also by individuals who were not aware of exactly what they were doing.

When you were young you used a

similar technique for the removal of pain. Remember when you would fall down and hurt your knee. You would grab your knee, take a deep breath, squeeze your muscles, then limp home where your mother would kiss it and make it well. Usually you really did feel better and most of the pain was gone. You were using three techniques for the removal or avoidance of pain: breath control, muscle control, and mind control. You used your breath to draw your body's healing powers to the area and to stop the nerve movement. You used your muscle to tighten the area and draw extra blood into it and relieve some of the pain. You used your mother's kiss as a mental affirmation that you no longer hurt.

An athlete is usually playing with some kind of pain. To get to be the best, he has to undergo much pain to perfect his game. It takes practice and a belief in his mind control to enable an athlete to throw away the pain. But more importantly it takes the desire of the athlete not to let an injury affect or stop his performance. Believe you can stop the pain and if you desire to stop the pain and to go on playing, you will certainly develop this technique.

PAIN-RELIEVING TECHNIQUES

Following are some techniques that can be applied to slight injuries that often occur in athletics. You can use these techniques for major injuries such as a broken bone or wounds, but we are concerned with injuries that are minor and that would allow an athlete to be unaffected by the pain so he could continue to play and perform at top level.

Joint Injuries—Slight Sprains and Jams

1. Take a deep breath and tighten the muscles that have been hurt. Now hold your breath while directing your mind to send your breath to the area that is hurt. (Of course you can't send air to the area—merely suggest to your mind that you are sending your breath with its healing properties to the injured area.)

2. Make circles, pointing away from the heart, around the affected area, not on the affected area. Rub around it about 5 to 10 times, then mentally take the pain into your fingertips and throw it away with a flick of your fingers—

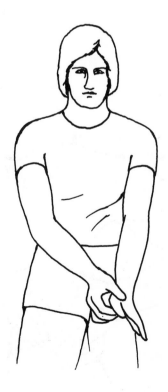

away from the body. (You can't actually throw away the pain, but you can give your mind and your body the auto-suggestion that you are throwing away the pain.)

3. Forget that you are injured and pay no more attention to any pain that may still be coming to the brain. Begin to reconcentrate very hard on the task or game at hand. Do not let the mind wander to the sensation of pain. Forget it; do not notice it. (Be like a man who works in a noisy factory and learns not to notice the noise after he has been there a while.) Don't worry that you may reinjure the area and your mind control may not let you notice the pain. The man in the factory who does not notice the noise immediately notices a strange sound; so, too, you will notice any further injury.

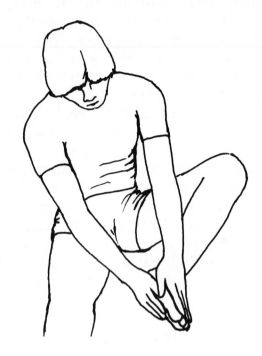

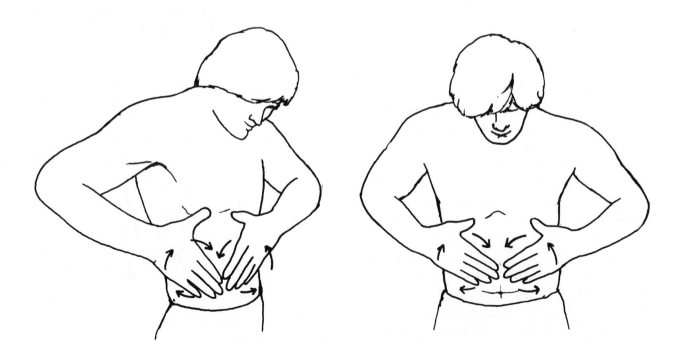

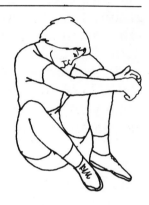

CHAPTER 7

Falling

Most coaches in America are not teaching proper methods of falling on the ground without being injured. I do not mean rolling forward, which is what most people think falling is. I am referring to getting your feet knocked out from under you and going four feet in the air and landing on your shoulder or neck, or being tackled or knocked down sideways and breaking your wrist, or slipping on the snow or ice and falling and injuring your tail bone or neck. These are examples of falls that athletes are constantly being exposed to and hurt from because they are not prepared to handle them. Players, coaches, and fans have expected a player to be injured when his feet are taken out from under him, or when he is thrown into the air—and if he isn't, it is a miracle.

There are only three basic ways a person can fall: forward, backward, or sideward. And there are proven, easy to learn techniques from judo that will reduce the chances of injury from a fall. Let us examine and practice techniques for each of the types of falls.

It is very important to practice these falls every day until they become second nature to you, because in real situations you fall suddenly and you often have only a split second to think. Your reflexes must be sharpened to the extent that you can fall in any direction with only the slightest notice. It may seem silly, but a good way to practice for these reflexes is to fall suddenly while you are walking, at your own discretion, and to practice and repractice your falls—especially the four-way falling techniques.

THE FORWARD FALL

There are two basic techniques for preventing injury in a forward fall. When the athlete has enough momentum or room, he should do a forward roll. When he must fall straight down, he should do a forward breakfall.

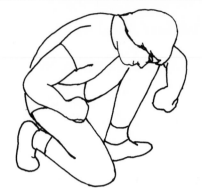

The Forward Roll

In this roll it is important to roll the shoulder over so that it does not hit the ground, and to have the same foot and same shoulder forward (your right foot with the right shoulder). Tuck the chin, avoid supporting your weight with your wrist, keep the body in a ball, and continue your rolling momentum until you are standing up again.

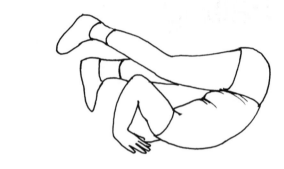

BEGINNER.

a. Squat down with the right knee and right shoulder forward.

b. Lean over, tuck the head, and roll the shoulder over forward.

c. Keep the body in a ball and land with one leg flat, the other straight ahead.

d. Roll up and stand.

Practice this at least 12 times from the right and left sides.

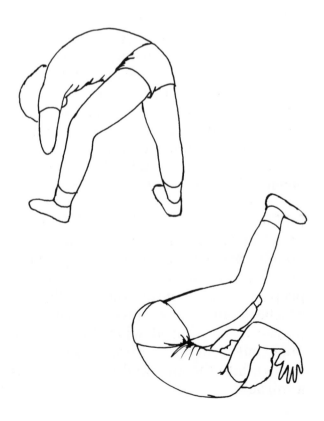

INTERMEDIATE.

a. Step forward with the right shoulder tucked down and the right leg forward.

b. Duck the head and bend over to the ground.

c. Curl the shoulder over and roll the body in a ball over the top of the shoulder.

d. Continue the roll until you are standing.

Practice this roll at least 12 times with each shoulder. Be careful not to put too much weight on the wrist during the roll and to tuck the head.

ADVANCED.

a. Have one partner kneel on the ground, very low.

b. Take a running start and jump over the partner.

c. While in the air tuck the shoulders and roll the body on the ground.

d. Continue the roll until you are standing up.

Add people on the ground until you can jump over three people. Do this at least 12 times. Practice your intermediate rolls every day during your practice session and before a game. It helps warm up the body and gets the blood circulating.

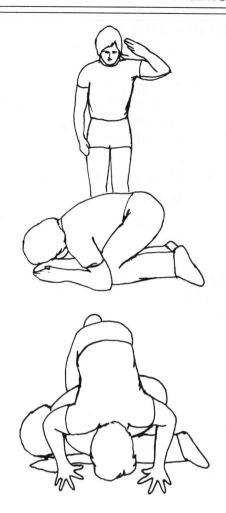

The Forward Breakfall

Sometimes a forward roll cannot be executed because of a wall or some other obstruction. Then it is necessary to do a forward breakfall to prevent injury. In this fall it is important to remember to absorb all the shock of the fall on the forearms and hands by slapping the ground very hard just before you hit it. Keep the head up and the back straight or slightly raised to keep the knees from hitting the ground.

BEGINNER.

a. Kneel on the ground with the hands in front of the body.

b. Fall forward, slapping the ground very hard before you hit.

c. Keep the buttocks off the ground and the head up.

d. Forcefully exhale your air as you hit.

Practice this fall at least 12 times.

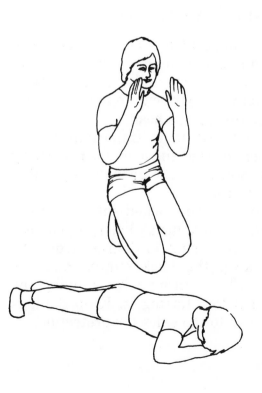

INTERMEDIATE.

a. Stand up with the arms held up in front of the body.

b. Bend the legs and slowly fall forward, slapping the ground very hard with the arms before hitting.

c. Keep the buttocks off the ground and the head up.

d. Yell and let your air out as you hit. Practice 12 times.

ADVANCED.

a. Stand straight up with the arms by the sides.

b. Jump forward as far as you can, slapping the ground with the hands before you hit.

c. Keep the trunk off the ground and the head up.

d. Yell and forcefully exhale your air to keep it from getting knocked out.

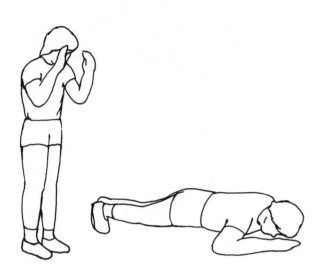

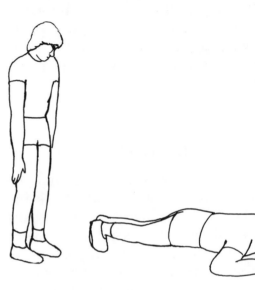

THE BACKWARD FALL

When an athlete finds his feet slipping out from under him or being knocked out from under him, he must fall backward without injuring his tail bone or hitting his head.

In this fall it is important to remember to bend the legs when slipping to get as close to the ground as possible before hitting.

Keep the chin tucked into the chest, slap with the arms as hard as you can, keeping the arms 45 degrees from the body; keep the back curved and the behind off the ground by slapping the ground before hitting it. Keep the legs crossed or to the sides for protection.

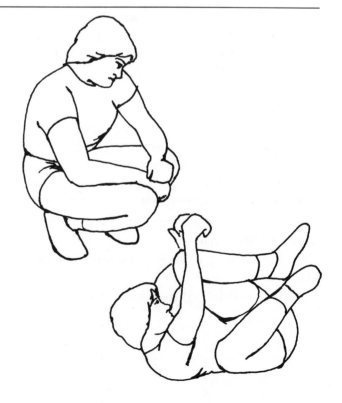

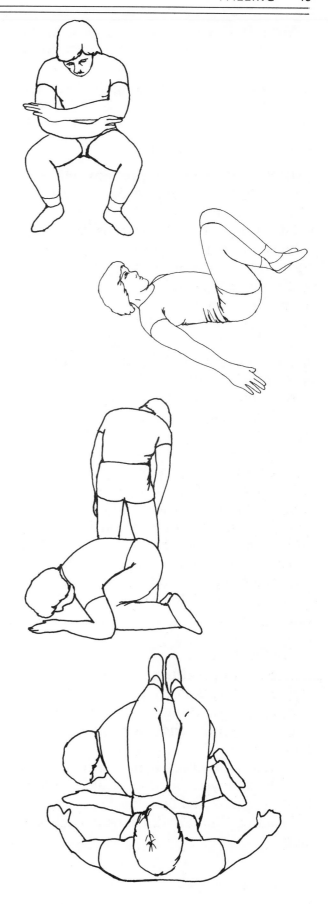

BEGINNER.

a. Sit on the ground and cross the arms in front.

b. Slowly lean backward slapping the ground very hard with the arms before your behind hits.

c. Keep the chin tucked into the chest; forcefully exhale the air.

d. Keep the back curved and the legs crossed or to the side.

Practice this fall 12 times.

INTERMEDIATE.

a. Stand up with the arms crossed in front of the body.

b. Step backward and begin to try to sit on the ground (an important point for it is much easier to fall from one foot than it is from five feet, and in most cases you are able to squat before you hit the ground).

c. Slap the ground very hard with the arms (notice how close the arms are to the body).

d. Keep the buttocks off the ground until last; keep the chin tucked into the chest so the head does not snap back and hit the ground.

e. Yell to let your air out, so it does not get knocked out of you.

Practice this fall 12 times.

ADVANCED.

a. Have a partner kneel on the ground very low.

b. Walk up briskly backward to the partner.

c. Fall over the partner and slap the ground before your buttocks or head hits.

d. Yell to let the air out so it does not get knocked out.

e. Continue to roll over and get back up.

Practice this fall 12 times.

Note: It is very easy to take a backward fall when one feels himself falling or has any type of warning. However, if one finds himself slipping on ice, for example, and falling backward, then he must think very fast so as to avoid hitting his coccyx or bumping his head. These fast reflexes come with practice.

THE SIDE BREAKFALL

Often the player will find himself falling to the sides, where care must be taken to avoid a shoulder injury or a wrist injury. The knee is particularly vulnerable in this position; proper falling and cover-up after falling can prevent many knee injuries.

The important points to remember: Never try to break the fall with your wrist; keep the legs straight or the knees bent to avoid knee injuries during or after the fall; slap the ground very hard; and exhale your air to keep it from being knocked out.

BEGINNER.

a. Kneel on the ground with the right leg in front of the left leg.

b. Slowly let yourself fall to the right, slapping the ground very hard with the right arm (note distance of arm from body); keep the knees bent slightly.

c. Keep the head off the ground.

Practice this fall 12 times to each side.

INTERMEDIATE.

a. Stand up with the right leg swinging across in front of the left.

b. Slap the ground very hard before you hit, keep the shoulder curled forward.

c. Keep the knees bent slightly.

d. Exhale your air forcefully to avoid having it knocked out.

Practice this fall 12 times to each side.

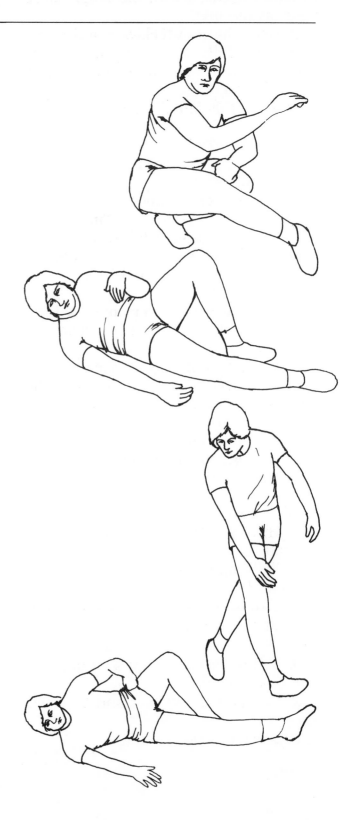

ADVANCED.

a. Have a partner kneel on the ground.

b. Run up to the partner and jump over him, landing on your side.

c. Slap the ground very hard, yell, and keep the knees bent slightly.

Practice this fall 12 times to each side.

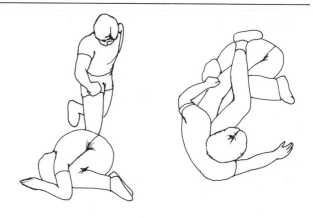

FALLING PRACTICE

The four-way fall is one of the most effective ways to practice your falls.

a. Jump forward into the forward breakfall; get up quickly.

b. Take a step and do a forward shoulder roll; roll up to your feet.

c. Take a step backward and fall backward; roll up to your feet.

d. Take a step sideways and fall to your side; cover and get up.

Do this 4 times, alternating sides on applicable falls.

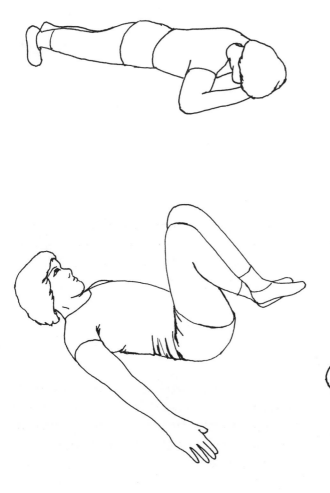

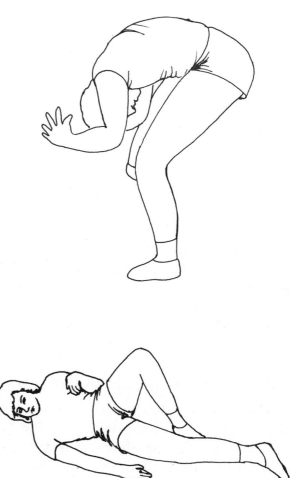

CHAPTER 8

The Knee

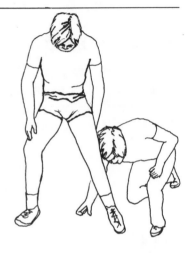

Although there is better equipment, better playing fields, better and stronger athletes, and better coaching, today there are more knee injuries than ever before. I believe that is because the knee is usually not worried about until it is too late. Not nearly enough emphasis is put on techniques that could prevent a knee injury.

PREVENTING KNEE INJURIES

The knee can be injured in the same three ways any other body part can be injured—by falling down and tearing and pulling its tendons or ligaments; by overstretching the ligaments or tendons; and by getting hit and breaking, tearing, or stretching it too much. Three simple but effective techniques can be used to help prevent most of the knee injuries.

Flexibility

It is important to get the knee flexible, but not to overstretch or tear the knee ligaments. So a simple rotary knee flexibility exercise is all that is needed. Bend down slightly and place both hands upon the knees. Make small circles to the right and to the left, about 10 in each direction. Now bounce up and down a few times and make 10 more circles to the right and left.

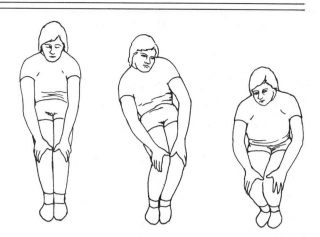

Ki in the Knee

It is quite possible to let someone run into or hit your knee when it is properly braced and you are using Ki to protect it. The knee must be slightly bent with the weight evenly displaced on both legs. As the blow comes you absorb most of the shock and control the knee in the direction you wish it to bend, not the direction the opponent wants it to bend. Practice the following.

a. Stand with the feet slightly wider than shoulder width and the weight centered.

b. Have a partner get down beside you and push his body weight against the knees.

c. Use your leg muscles to hold the knee tight; use breath control by breathing out very sharply to concentrate the muscles and control or focus the mind.

d. Shift your weight over to the opposite leg and begin to collapse forward with the knee being hit, bending the knee and consciously pulling it up to bend. *Note:* Do not place a lot of weight on the ball of your foot. That would decrease your control over the position of the fall.

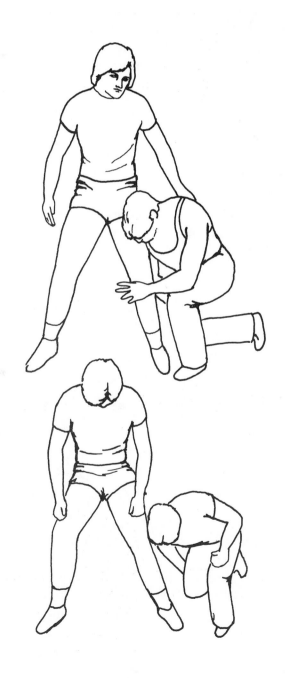

Falling to Protect the Knees

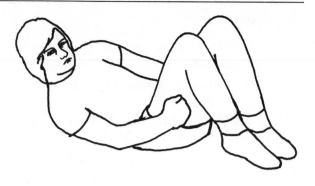

When you are hit on the knees or when you are falling in any position, BEND THE KNEES and try to tuck them up; in other words fold your legs. You cannot have your knee injured if your legs are bent in half.

Sometimes the knee is injured after you have fallen because someone may fall on it or step on it. To avoid this remember that the play is not over just because you are on the ground. When you are on the ground, immediately bend both knees up to your chest. If you find yourself with one leg out and caught so you can't bend it, then roll over on your stomach. If you can't bend your leg or roll over on your stomach, then try to lift the leg and bend it up.

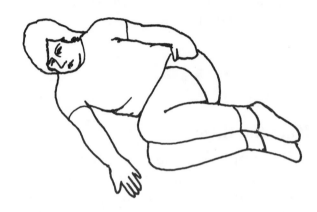

Continue to think about preventing injuries even when you are on the ground. Immediately take a look at your knees and bend them as quickly as you can or roll over. Many times knee injuries can be prevented by this technique.

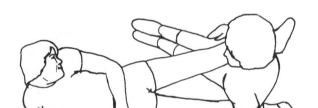

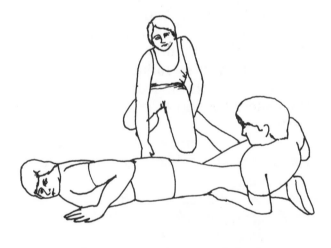

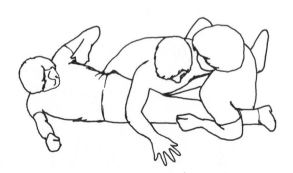

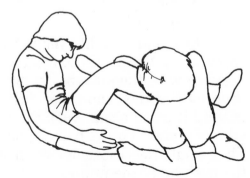

CHAPTER 9

Relaxation

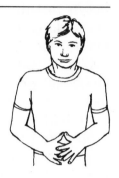

The ability to relax cannot be overemphasized and can be defined for our use to mean the ability to leave the game out of your body, but keep it in your mind. Too many coaches and players lose points, and sometimes get ulcers, because they cannot control their tempers or attitudes during the game situation. They have let their reactions be determined by the actions of other people, referees, or players. Therefore, they find themselves like puppets on a string—ranting and raving, or awkward and clumsy—because they have destroyed the delicate relationship between the body and the mind. They have let their emotions have too much control over their actions; because of that they have lost their style, poise, and grace. (Some examples: The coach in the ball game who runs up and down the sidelines, kicking the ground and the players and screaming and shouting at the referee; the player who can't make a shot because he is so nervous and anxiety ridden; the player who jumps offsides several times or who starts fights at the slightest provocation.)

The problem with these people is that they have lost control of their bodies by letting their minds become confused and disoriented. The mind cannot think of two things at once and do a good job on either one. You must have a calm mind if you want to make the shot, or to think the play out. Your mind directs your muscles to perform as they have been conditioned, but if your mind is racing between being upset and making the shot (being angry and being relaxed), then the muscles receive contradictory information. Rather than performing as programmed, they become uncoordinated. The brain becomes confused by the huge influx of emotional stimuli; it can't reason intelligently or perform adequately and begins to send out all kinds of emergency signals to the body. Because the mind cannot distinguish between a vividly imagined event and an actual occurrence, when you begin to think angry, your brain interprets danger and sends out the appropriate body responses. Your adrenaline starts to be released, thereby causing the blood pressure to go up, the heart to beat faster, the stomach to stop digesting and begin secreting acid, the eyes to dilate, and the muscles to become jerky and tensed. So your body is prepared for attack or defense, and when none comes the damage is irreversible. No one is easier to handle than a man who has gone so crazy with anger that he is like a wild man; he obviously can't perform his primary function in the game. Having such a player on your side probably causes others to perform badly also. Ulcers and lost games, fights and lost friends are just some of the results of the inability to relax.

Any great athletic performance seems effortless because the athlete has practiced and practiced until he has programmed his body for the appropriate response. He has learned to keep his mind calm and to relax while performing, thereby conserving his energy and assuring a longer and better performance. He is like a work of art, graceful and beautiful to look at, because he has achieved harmony between his body and mind.

A great coach is the same thing. He has learned to teach and train his team with patience, kindness, and understanding. He has confidence in his team and his coaching staff. He knows that they will do the best they can, and that the game is not the time to change previously conditioned responses or to try to do a coaching job that should have been done in practice sessions. So he remains calm and relaxed on the sidelines and usually winds up winning. Of course there are coaches who become involved to a great extent and are also winners, but they don't last as long and generally pay for their involvement with ulcers and loss of friends and support. No one likes you when you are upset—especially your own body. So let's practice a form of relaxation that takes only three minutes and can be as beneficial as one hour of sleep.

RELAXATION TECHNIQUE

Relaxing

Lie on the floor with the feet together and the palms face down at the sides. Look straight up and do not move the eyes. This is important. Now take a deep breath, hold it for a second and tighten the feet. Now relax and exhale. As you do, say to yourself, "relax; my feet are relaxed." Now take a deep breath and tighten the calves. Hold the tension for a second. As you release the breath say gently to yourself, "my calves are relaxed." Take another deep breath and tighten the thighs. Hold it for a second. As you release the breath, relax the thighs. Your legs are now completely relaxed. You no longer wish to move your legs. You could move your legs, but you no longer wish to move them. Take a deep breath into your stomach; hold it. As the air leaves your stomach, relax your stomach. Now breathe deeply into your lungs. As the air leaves your lungs, relax your chest and let your breath become very subtle and soft. Now breathe and tighten the arms and hands. Hold the tension a second, then relax. As the breath leaves, your arms become very relaxed. Your entire body is now very relaxed and you feel as if you are floating on a cloud, very calm and very relaxed. Take a breath and tighten your neck and shoulders. Hold it and as you let your breath out relax your neck area. Now take a breath and make a large frown, an ugly face. Now relax and breathe out; relax your face more and more until your jaw almost drops open. Your entire body is now completely relaxed; you feel extremely calm and relaxed. The only thing left to relax are your eyes. Gently close your eyes. You should immediately start dreaming.

Just let your mind roam and relax; dream of soft and nice things. Imagine you are floating on a raft in a calm lake, or sailing on a cloud. Relax and feel the air flow through your body; relax and dream. Relax and dream. Let the mind float from one thought to the next, paying no special attention to any thought. Just watch them come and go in the mind like you see cars come and go on the highway. Relax and think of beautiful things. Think of nature, music, art, love. Relax and feel yourself floating.

Now when one wishes to come out of this relaxed atmosphere, one should not just jump up. Gently open the eyes and take a deep breath; move the fingertips and the toes; breathe again and move the arms and the legs; breathe again and bend the arms and legs; move the hips. Now take the arms and rub the back of the neck and calmly sit up and relax in a meditative posture for a few more seconds. You will feel very relaxed and quite calm and refreshed. This is truly a valuable way of letting an athlete relax and should be used by all serious students.

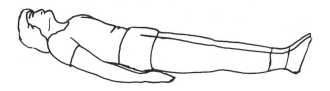

Three minutes of this relaxation is better for the body than one hour of sleep because it calms the nerves, refreshes the spirit, and soothes the mind. It is fast and simple to do and can be used after a workout or running. (Three minutes of sitting on the side of the track with the head between the legs trying to regain the breath after running does very little to relax you, but three minutes of this exercise does wonders.)

You can do this exercise lying down; it is very helpful to those who have trouble going to sleep. You can also do it standing up or sitting on the sidelines during the game. As a coach, just take a few deep breaths and tighten the muscles just as if you were lying down. In a few breaths you will begin to become calm and feel more relaxed. Just close your eyes for a few seconds and suggest to yourself a few pleasant thoughts. Your mind should become calm and relaxed, and soon your performance as a coach and player will be at its strongest point.

Breathing

The mind cannot be relaxed and calm when the body is breathing fast and furiously. So the necessity of regaining control over your breath as soon as possible after exertion is very important. Often when we run, we begin to experience anoxia—we get too much blood pumping too much oxygen and lose the delicate balance between good and bad air in our bodies. So we must use our mind to control our breathing, to slow it and allow the oxygen, carbon dioxide stages to be equalized.

Deep breathing, or circular breathing, should be used to assure your muscles of an adequate supply of air when you find yourself breathing too fast after exertion.

Stand with the feet shoulder width apart and touch the hands together in front of the body. Begin the breath very slowly and easily as the arms are lifted up in a clockwise circle around the head and down the sides of the body; continue to breathe in air during the entire circle. After doing this three times, you will feel refreshed and have a more adequate air supply to necessary muscles.

As you practice doing this exercise, you will learn to control your breathing to be able to get more benefit from the circular breathing. It is the fastest and easiest way to regain the proper breathing control after running or strong physical exertion.

The breath plays an important part in the relaxation of the body. Often it is the breath that determines the body's responses, not the body that determines the breath's reaction. In other words, you are not breathing fast because you have been running; you are able to run because you are able to breathe quickly in order to supply the additional oxygen

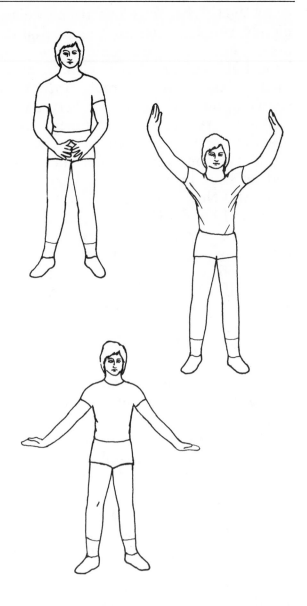

requirements to the body. If you could not breathe well, you would be asthmatic and unable to perform any vigorous exercise.

Your breath is the most important thing in your body. It is the only thing that you cannot consciously deprive yourself of. You can poke your eyes out, kill yourself for love, bust your ear drums listening to loud music, deprive yourself of food, but you cannot hold your breath until you suffocate and you cannot let someone else suffocate you. Your body will not just relax and let itself be deprived of air. You will do anything to anyone when the need for air becomes dire for your survival.

The breath plays a very important part in relaxation because it plays a large part in the control of our body's reactions to certain events. For example, we have already noted that you could not run if you were not able to breathe fast and deep enough to supply the additional oxygen requirement needed by the body. When you are angry, your breath becomes short and fast like when you are running. But when you are sleeping, your breath becomes slow and deep and relaxed and so does your mind. You cannot be breathing slow and deep and relaxed if you are angry or if you are upset. When you breathe calmly, your mind and muscles respond calmly. The calm breath can still the mind and the nerves.

Practice the following exercises which were developed centuries ago by people who understood the importance of the breath as a factor in self-understanding and in mind and body control.

COUNTING THE BREATHS. Sit in a meditative position (see Chapter 10) and take a few deep breaths to calm the mind. Now begin to concentrate only on the breath as it comes in and as it leaves the body. Try to clear the mind of all outside thoughts and concentrate only on the incoming and outgoing breaths. When you begin to breathe in, think only of the number One or only of this being your first breath. Let no other thoughts enter your mind but the number One. Continue to concentrate on this number all the way through the breath and as you begin to breathe out; continue to think and concentrate only on the number One. Then as you begin your next breath think and concentrate only on the number Two. Clear the mind of all other thoughts and think only of the number Two as you breathe in and as you breathe out. Continue to do this slow breathing and concentration up to the number Ten. Keep the mind calm, and concentrate only on the numbers.

In a very few seconds you will see the difficulty of clearing the mind. Thoughts will begin to float up and your mind will become distracted from your primary purpose of thinking and seeing only the numbers. But do not become discouraged. This is an exercise and technique that can take years of practice to do perfectly. The mind is always full of extra thoughts, and you must practice trying to calm it just as you would practice trying to learn a new skill—over and over again with patience and a calm and resolved manner. You cannot still the mind by being angry at it for thinking other thoughts; you cannot calm the mind by tightening the muscles. Just relax and try to concentrate the mind only on the breath.

Gradually you will be able to think only of the numbers. However, if you are having great difficulty in visualizing the numbers, then perhaps the visualization of colors will be easier for you. When you breathe in, think only of the color red through the entire breath, then of the color blue, then green, then orange, then black, then white, then yellow, then brown, then purple, and finally pink (or you can use any order you wish).

You should perform this counting exercise every day for at least a few weeks until you have begun to gain some control of your mind. Practice should only take a few minutes, up to five, so you should always be able to find the time to practice. Eventually, you may want to do the exercise more often for the relaxing effects it has on the mind and body. You may do it as often or as little as you wish. You can do it whenever you find yourself getting upset. Remember how your mother told you to count to ten if you were angry. The same effect is achieved now but you are adding the effect of the slow and easy breathing to calm the nerves and soothe the mind.

CONTROLLING THE BREATH. This exercise trains you in the voluntary control of the breath by the conscious will of the mind. You will not be allowing the body to breathe normally but will be trying to force it to breathe as the mind wishes.

Sit in the meditative position and close the eyes. Take a few deep breaths to calm the mind. Slowly begin to breathe in for the count of 10; count each number silently to yourself. Now hold your breath without pressing down or lifting your shoulders up for the count of 10. Now begin to breathe out for the count of 10, trying to make the out-breathing slow and controlled and not breathing out all the air at the beginning of the out-breath. Immediately after you have breathed out for 10, begin to breathe in again for the count of 10. Hold it in for 10 and out for 10. Do this exercise 10 times. You will find that you may start to sweat and that you really have to use a lot of muscles and mind control to stop your body from breathing in or out too quickly. This is an excellent form of breathing control; the benefits are numerous. It teaches the mind great strength and begins to reconfirm to the muscles the power of the mind over them. It produces a body heat, and so can be used if you are cold; and it strengthens the breath control by the actual controlling of the breathing movement. You can consider yourself

exceptional if you can breathe in for 30 seconds, hold it for 30 seconds, and breathe out for 30 seconds—10 times. This shows a true mastery of the breath and a great deal of muscle and mind control. Do this exercise daily for a few weeks until you have been able to do all 10 breaths in the correct count. Thereafter you may do it as often as you wish for the benefits it provides the muscles.

FOLLOWING THE BREATH. The purpose of this exercise is to transcend the mind—to concentrate only on the breath as it fills the body and the lungs and to follow it as it comes and goes in and out. This is a very soothing and relaxing form of breathing and the benefits are long lasting and comforting.

Sit in the meditative position and close the eyes. Take a few deep breaths to calm the mind and relax the nerves. Now as you begin to breathe in, try to let all other thoughts leave the mind except following the breath as it goes through your nostrils, down your throat and fills your lungs, then is dispersed to the various parts of your body. Follow it as it returns up your throat and out your nostrils and into the air. Try to imagine a golden string being attached to your lungs that comes out of you as you breathe the air out and comes back into the lungs as you breathe in. Let your mind remain calm; follow the breath softly and easily. Soon you will begin to feel the body become filled with air, and you will begin to feel very calm and relaxed, very soothed and light. The breath will fill your mind and your body and you will begin to feel as light as your breath itself. Do this exercise as long as you feel light and are able to concentrate on following the breaths. It is very soothing and relaxing. Do this exercise any time you are upset or any time you wish to feel truly relaxed.

CHAPTER 10

The Tiger Eye

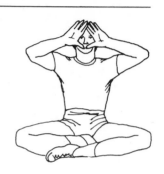

The "Tiger Eye" is a term that we will use to mean peripheral vision, or the ability to see everything that is surrounding you without moving the eyes or the head. This technique is very valuable in most sports because it increases awareness and performance. If you can see everything that surrounds you, the chances of your throwing an interception, or missing a tackle or shot, are greatly reduced.

MEDITATION

The Half Lotus Position

There are as many different positions for meditation (or concentration on a specific thought towards a specified goal) as there are forms of meditation. All have their benefits but some of them are difficult to do, so we will use a simple but effective position, called in yoga the half lotus position.

Sit on the floor with the legs crossed in front of the body. Place the right leg in first and cross the left leg in front of that. Strive to keep the knees as near the ground as possible and the back, spine, and neck in a straight line. Rock back and forth and gently to the sides to assure you are sitting up straight. Place the arms on the tops of the knees with the palms up. This helps to stabilize and balance the back. You may feel uncomfortable in this position. That is because you are not flexible enough. To improve flexibility do the stretches found earlier in the book, but if you are not flexible because you have not been doing the stretches long enough, you may modify the position so that you are grabbing the knees or even putting the legs straight out. You may even sit in a straight-backed chair while you are learning your flexibility.

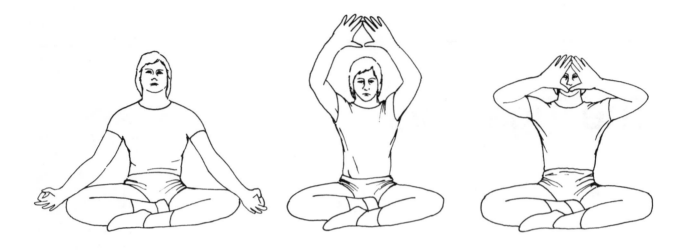

PRACTICING THE TIGER EYE

After one has assumed the meditative position, he should fix the gaze of his eyes directly ahead and on one point. The hands should be held above the head to start with, the fingers forming a triangle, and then slowly brought down to in front of the eyes. The eyes should be fixed in a gaze upon one area and should no longer move. The hands should then be placed on the knees, palms up with the thumb and forefinger interjoined. Now the Tiger Eye should be practiced.

You will find upon investigation that when the eyes are looking straight ahead and not focusing too sharply on one particular object that all the field of vision can be seen. But if you move your eyes side to side very fast or move your head quickly, then everything becomes blurred and you cannot see things clearly—just as a good hunter looks only at the trees and notices the slightest movement, not at the individual limbs and seeing only those limbs. Just imagine that the field of vision is like a small painting. You can see all of the painting clearly but not if you are moving your head or your eyes from side to side. So try to get in the habit of moving the whole body when you move the eyes. That way you keep the vision clear and the body in position to react. (For example, if you look out the corner of your eye, you can see someone about to hit you, but your body would not be in a very strong position for defending yourself. It is better to turn the whole body to look.)

You can practice the Tiger Eye while walking. Just look straight ahead when you walk and do not move the eyes. You will see all the people coming and going around you; you will see movement to the right and left. You will feel calm and hear things you have not noticed before; you will be practicing your peripheral vision, and you will be soothing your nerves and calming your mind.

Looking and Listening

Let us assume you are looking at a football field during a game and you are standing in the middle of the field facing the goal line. Without moving your eyes you can see the following things: You can see the goal posts and the end zone; you can see the stripes on the field and the grass, and the colors of the grass; you can see the sidelines, and the benches full of other players on the sidelines; you can see the players on the playing field, all of the players, and you can see the sky; you can see the lights around the stadium and the fans in the seats around the stadium; you can see the players directly beside you and across from you. In other words, you can see everything—in front of you, on the side of you, above you, and below your feet.

Now listen, you can hear the crowd. You can hear the sports announcer. You can hear the coach and players yelling on the sidelines. You can hear the quarterback and the players on the field talking, and even walking or hitting each other on the plays. You can see everything and you can hear everything going on around you. This is total awareness, total visual and sensory awareness. You cannot be surprised by a clip, or scared by a yell of another player. You are aware, just like the tiger is aware in the jungle. Yet you are relaxed and ready to move in any direction at any time, just like the tiger in the jungle.

The "Tiger Eye" is most useful for foul shooting, quarterbacks, safeties, linebackers, and coaching. All good coaches are able to look at the play and see the whole play unfolding at once, not just one player at a time. So a spotter who uses this technique will be a more effective spotter because he will be able to see the whole field and the whole play at once.

The "Tiger Eye" enables you to hear all the sounds and see all the sights around you. A good player is not drawn off sides by the change in the quarterback's cadence or inflection, and a good player does not lose concentration when the crowd boos him or is screaming at him or the team. He is just concentrating on the shot or the game. He hears the noise but is not distracted by it.

Visualizations

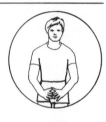
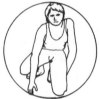

Visualization is the conscious action of forming mental pictures in the mind. These pictures can be used for learning, for relaxation, and for improvement of techniques.

LEARNING THROUGH VISUALIZATIONS

As we have noted previously, the mind interprets and integrates the thoughts or sensations that occur and translates them into visual concepts or pictures inside the mind. But the mind cannot distinguish between a vividly imagined event and an actual occurrence. Therefore the mind can be programmed to believe certain concepts and ideas; when the mind internalizes or really believes these concepts, the body will tend to find ways to make them come true. (For example, if you believe you will be an All-American, your body will be given the determination to achieve the physical skills necessary to become an All-American.)

The body cannot perform any skill that the mind cannot see the body performing. You cannot be a great tennis player if you cannot see yourself making great tennis shots in your mind. You must be able to see every muscular position that your body would be in to actually make the great shots.

If we would like to use visualization

for learning, let us say for learning a new play in football, we can use the following exercises:

Meditational Imagination

Sitting in the meditative position, close the eyes and imagine you are about to perform the play you are trying to learn. Where are your feet supposed to be as you come up and get down on the line? Who is to the right of you, the left of you? Who is across from you? Where are you supposed to make him go? What noises will you be hearing at the start of the play? At the snap of the ball, what is the first movement of your feet? Where are your shoulders and arms supposed to be? Who is beside you now? What is the new position of the man facing you? As you move toward him, how are your feet supposed to be? What is his movement? Where is the ball carrier? What noises are surrounding you? As you make contact, where are your arms and legs supposed to be? How far back and to what direction are you supposed to move him? Take yourself in your mind step by intricate step through the entire play. Do this several times, each time adding new points to your movement or blocking that you may have forgotten before. This is an excellent and effective way to practice and learn new plays, or improve on old ones. You can do this at home, while lying in bed, while walking, anywhere.

Writing It Down

Write down on a piece of paper all the various aspects of the play. What is your job? Where are you supposed to be at the snap, at the first movement? Who are you blocking and to where? For how long? Who is beside you, to the right and left? When is the ball snapped and how long does the play last? Write down in intricate detail the entire play. Read it to your teammates for group discussion. Ask the coach what was left out and how the play could be improved. You are using techniques of visualization when you write the movements down.

To the Coach

Have the player take you through the play step by step, as if he were the coach. You take his place in the line and make the same mistakes and errors he previously made, or new ones to see how he can correct you. The player will learn more by teaching than he does by playing. He will have to visualize the play in his mind and tell you what you are doing wrong or right, so he will be reinforcing the learning.

Visualizations of Winning

It is not enough merely to say "We are number 1." The player and the coaches must see themselves as being number 1 because they see themselves beating the tough teams. If you want to use visualizations to get the mind to believe that you can beat the tough teams and that you can be number 1, practice the following exercise.

Assume the meditative position and close the eyes. Now vividly imagine that you are at the ball park just as the game is about to be over with your toughest rival. Use all your senses in the visualization. Hear the roar of the crowd, smell the air, feel your uniform on your back and your muscles after a hard game, touch the ground and the players around you, taste the sweat dripping down your forehead from a hard-fought battle. See the field and the scoreboard, and see your team ahead with just one minute to go. Begin to watch the clock as you see the other team hopelessly trying to stop your drive, but it's too late because you have three downs left and they have no timeouts. Count the seconds down on the clock as you listen to the fans begin to count with you. Feel the excitement in the air, smell the excitement, begin to get excited and jump up and down, shaking hands and slapping the backs of the other players. At last, the clock is down to 10 seconds and the crowd is starting to gather around the field—3, 2, 1, bang! The game is over and you jump for joy. You have beaten the best team in the league. Vividly imagine this every night before you go to sleep, practice it as a team months before the big game, internalize the belief, and use the visualization again and again. Your mind will come to believe it and accept it as a true fact, and the body will have the desire and determination to practice and the courage and skill to keep on trying. The body will not make any mistakes in the big game, thus assuring the victory that you have by now become confident of in your mind.

Visualizations for Relaxation

Have you ever been to the Alps, or Buckingham Palace in England, or the Amazon in Brazil? Probably not, but in your mind, because of the wonders of TV and movies, you have formed visual pictures of these places and it is just like you were really there. The ability to form these visual pictures can be used as a method of relaxation to help you go to sleep and have pleasant dreams. Lie down and take a few deep breaths to calm the mind. Then slowly let your mind drift over some pleasant thoughts and scenes like the mountains, the lakes, or the forest. As one of these thoughts begins to get clear in the mind, softly begin to linger there and to visualize yourself standing in the middle of the mountain beauty. Feel the soft breeze on your face, and smell the clean fresh air. Look around you at the wonders of nature, and hear the beautiful sounds of life that surround you. Begin to hear soft and lovely music as you continue to enjoy the sights. Perhaps now you have been joined by a loved one you would like to share this scene with. Talk to this person as if she (or he) were there, and touch and feel her as if she were there. Let your mind float and your thoughts expand with the scenery until in your mind you feel as though you were really there. After a few minutes you will become very calm and relaxed and begin to truly dream or sleep.

CHAPTER 12

Goal Setting

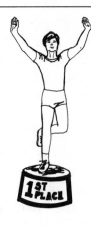

Many people think of goal setting as daydreaming because they have hazy goals, or goals that are unrealistic for them to achieve in the foreseeable future. Such things as being a millionaire or being President. You can be all things if you believe in yourself, develop a sensible and workable plan for achieving the results you desire, and have such a burning desire and determination to achieve your goals that no person or no thing will stop you. Goals to us will not mean far off daydreams. Goals are plans, feasible and workable plans, that are actively being pursued in an organized and predetermined fashion.

Why is it necessary to have goals, you might say. Well suppose you had a child and you wanted to teach him to throw and catch a baseball. That is your goal or your plan. In order to do it in the most effective and fastest way, it is logical that you develop his skills little by little. You would have a purpose in each thing you show him as a development of the skill of throwing and catching a baseball. He can't throw the ball with either hand; he must specialize and practice on just one. He can't just throw the ball up, or backward; he must throw it toward a target. The reward comes when he hits his target. If you just give the child a ball and say go and play, he will develop improper or inadequate skills and usually become frustrated and give up on the sport. But if you have a plan for teaching him the skills and time for him to practice the skills, then the goal of throwing a baseball is achieved in the fastest time and with the most effective results.

The same thing is true of an athlete. He can't just have a vague goal and just want to play football. He must want to learn to play a definite position, he must acquire definite skills in order to excel at that position, and he must have a plan of action for achieving or practicing these skills. If he just goes out and tries every position and never learns or practices the skills necessary to excel in that position, he is a man without goals; and he will get nowhere in football or life.

PLANS

Everyone has goals. Unfortunately most people are working toward someone else's goals. Especially in sports too many players are just working on the goals the coaches have for them. So they go through their careers never achieving the potential greatness within themselves. If the player would make it his goal to become an All-American and map out in intricate detail the problems he has to overcome, the solutions to these problems, the time he has to achieve his goal, and the progressive steps in achieving them, then there is no reason he cannot become an All-American.

There are many things the player should take into consideration in his becoming an All-American. What special skills does he have to achieve to be All-American? How fast does he have to be able to run to be an All-American? What should his muscular strength be? How much time should he practice a day, and on what skills? How many blocks, tackles, assists, etc., will he need to make in a game? How many yards will he need to gain, or stop the other team from gaining? Does he need the cooperation of other players or the coaches? How many seasons does he have left to play and when can he realistically expect to make the All-American team?

These and other questions must be answered by the player in detail before he begins his quest for becoming an All-American. After he has answered these questions, he must begin to write a plan of action. He must write down and organize himself to the smallest detail for what he needs to achieve and when he will practice each day to achieve these goals. Then he must begin working on his plan, every day without fail, determined and persistent in the pursuit of his goal. If the player remains resolved and keeps his vigorous practice schedule up, there is no reason he cannot make All-District, All-State, and then All-American.

The coaches should also have goals and intricate plans of action for the members of the team. Such things as: How many players should be able to bench press 300 pounds and run the forty-yard dash in four seconds? How many players of each position should they pursue in recruitment? How many victories do they need to win the conference? How many fumbles would be acceptable each game? How many yards should the defense allow? How many field goals should they get in each specific game? How many touchdowns should they get in each game? How many points should they get? How many points should each player get?

What does the assistant coach expect from each player? What does the coach expect from each assistant coach?

These and many other questions the coaches should answer in detail, so they know exactly what they have to get in each game and from each player and under what situations. If they are not sure of certain points, they should find out exactly what they expect. Then the coach should write a plan of action and begin to follow it religiously day by day, hour by hour. His time should be devoted to and organized such that he is always making definite progress on his personal and team goals.

PRACTICE

Often the optimal effects are not achieved during the practice session. Every practice session, however, can be extremely productive and rewarding if the players and coaches learn to relate to this story.

The Japanese women's volleyball team practices 365 days a year, three hours a day—and the women are never heard to complain or ever miss a practice. Each practice session is done as if it were the one before the big game, and each player gives 110 percent at each practice. That is why they are number 1 in the world. But what attitudes are in the minds of the women as they practice? The answer may surprise you. If you were to walk up to one of the women and ask her, "How long have you been practicing, when do you get a break, why don't you get a day off?" or any of a dozen other questions that seem to fill the minds of the press and the fans, the answer would be, "I'll be right with you, right now I am playing volleyball." Not "I have been playing for 234 days without a break, I am sick of playing, the coach is mean, I never get a day off, I have been playing two hours and only have an hour to go, thank God."

Just "I am playing volleyball." You see, the Japanese women have learned to master the art of concentration; because of that their minds are only on the game of volleyball, only on the point at hand—not on yesterday's mistakes, tomorrow's practice, or next year's practice. Not on the coach, but only on the game at that very minute. Extreme, intense, complete concentration on the present moment, on one specific thing. To make the point. Now! So in your practice session, or your game, your mind should not be wandering on when session will be over, or on the last play, or on how big the guy is you're trying to block or tackle, or on how many games you have left, or on your girl friend. You should play one play at a time and use all your concentration and energy and skill to do what you are supposed to be doing in that one particular play. Block that guy, tackle that guy, throw to that guy—only concentrate on that one fact. If you blow it, forget it and begin to concentrate on the next play—one play at a time, one tackle at a time, and keeping your mind concentrated just like the volleyball team.

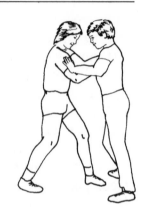

CHAPTER 13

Explosive Power in Movement

No other sport in the world generates as much explosive power through movement as does Karate. Weight lifters have a lot of strength, but not the kind that combines speed and agility with power. Karate has developed techniques that enable people of slight build and small muscle mass to hit so hard and kick so powerfully that they are able to smash through bricks, wood, or bodies. They get that power and you can get it by practicing the exercises in this chapter.

HIP MOVEMENT

Most athletes use only the strength of one muscle part. In other words, a boxer hits you with his arms, a weight lifter pushes with his legs or arms, a football player hits you with his elbow or shoulder. They have not learned the tremendous amount of power that can be generated by the use of the entire body, especially the snapping and thrusting of the hips, to generate explosive power. Muscle alone will not provide enough power. Imagine a very heavy sledgehammer. The power potential is enormous, but it is so heavy that you cannot swing it with enough speed to generate any force or power. So the huge potential power of the sledgehammer essentially is wasted. The same is true of many athletes. They have tremendous potential for power but they

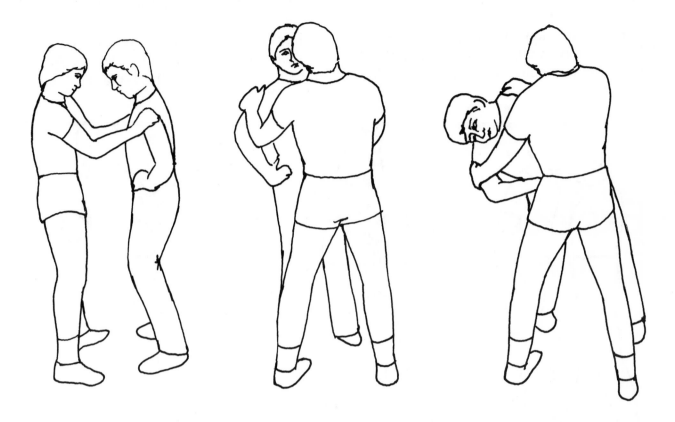

reduce their effectiveness many times because they are too slow or use only one body part to generate this power. The power that can be generated by a body is equal to this formula: $P = S \times M \times BM$ or Power equals Speed of the movement times the Muscular strength behind it times the unified Body Movement at the time of impact. So we must work to develop speed, coordination, and muscle; we must use all three simultaneously and focus them at the point and instant of contact.

Weight Shifting Exercise

Have the partners stand facing each other. One partner places his arms on the shoulder of the other. Now without moving his arms any wider than they already are, one partner must generate a whipping action of the hips and throw the partner to the side. It is easy to see that if one tries to throw him to the side with just his arm strength, he cannot do it. Do this at least 15 times with each partner. Practice every day until mastered.

One-Inch Punch

Using the hips as a power generator and locking the arm in the manner we have learned from the unbendable arm techniques, it is possible to develop devastating power from only one inch away from the partner.

Have the partners stand facing each other with one slightly to the side. One places his elbow against the chest of the partner. Without drawing his elbow back, but by swinging and snapping up from his legs and through his hips, he explodes his speed and force through his elbow and knocks the partner backward.

Perform this exercise at least 15 times. Continue daily until you have mastered this hip explosiveness.

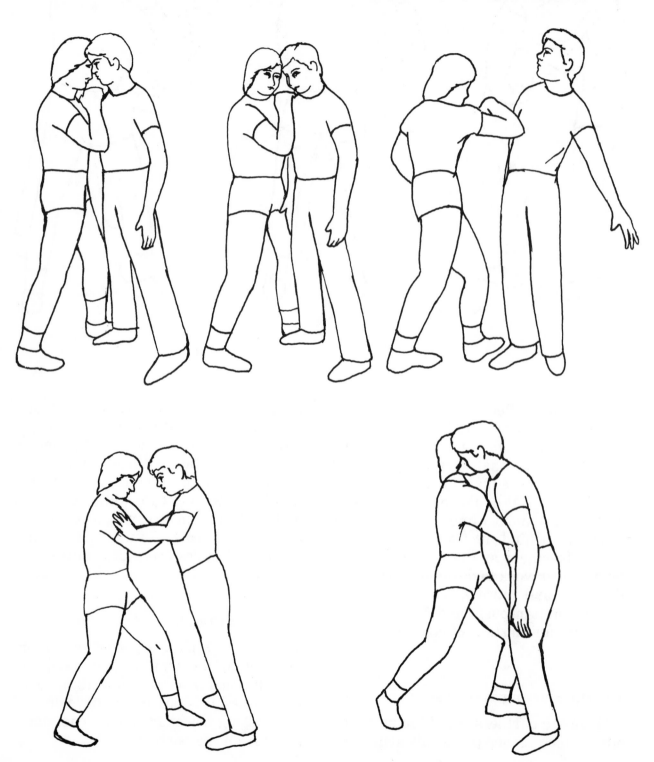

The Elbow Smash

Often in football the players will hit an opponent in the chest or block him by using their elbows to swing up and hit the chest area. There will be a loud noise but usually not much damage. This is because once the elbows are the level of the shoulder, they have almost no strength left in them to raise them any higher. So to generate the most power from this blow, one should not lift his elbows any higher than the middle of the chest and should use his legs and hips for the power generation to explode through the opponent. Simply snap through the legs and pop the hips up, keeping the elbows locked and arms unbendable, and the force will be powerful and explosive.

Often just one elbow is used to hit the opponent, but this elbow loses most of its power if it is used simply as an arm and shoulder swing. If you will snap the hips and thrust the body weight into the strike, keeping the elbow near the body, you will be able to explode through the opponent and create much more power.

To generate the most explosive power, begin to analyze your body positions when you are hitting someone or something and try to get as much of the hip movement and speed plus muscle into the blow as possible. Always exhale your air forcefully at the instant of impact. This allows for more muscle contraction and increased concentration with more power.

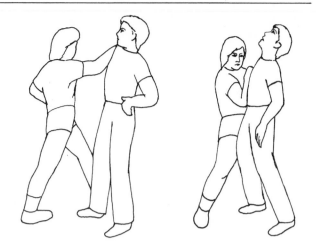

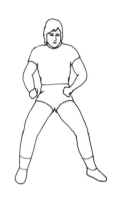

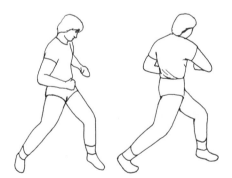